# ESSENTIAL GUIDE ON PCOS DIET TO HELP PEOPLE LOSE WEIGHT

———

Elena Miller

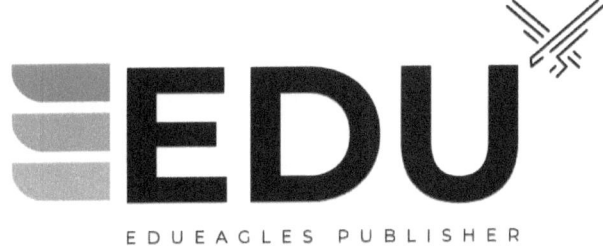

EDUEAGLES PUBLISHER

## INTRODUCTION

You will see a number of PCOS diets being advertised online, and it can be difficult to decide which one to follow. Like all diets, there isn't one definitive program that will be effective at the expense of all the others, but you should be on the look out for certain elements within the program to make sure it's suitable for losing weight with PCOS and not likely to cause your body more harm than good.

The most important thing to remember is that once you commit to following a healthy eating program you stick to it. This can be especially important when you have PCOS, as weight loss may not occur as quickly as it does for other women and you can often hit a plateau or "sticking point". If you are becoming frustrated with not losing weight, remind yourself you are eating for health, not just weight loss, and that by following a PCOS diet you are preventing further health problems in the future.

Another important element to look for and avoid is promises of fast weight loss, after which you can return to your old eating habits. This will result in yo-yo dieting, and ultimately will mean the weight being put back on and you finding it harder to lose weight the next time, potentially putting your body at risk of other health issues.

When you are assessing PCOS diets you should look for how they propose to combat Insulin Resistance. Research shows that many women with PCOS have Insulin Resistance or are likely to develop it. This means they need a diet that keeps blood sugar and insulin levels steady. Apart from the short-term effects of this, which include increased weight gain, lack of energy and increased hunger, it can eventually lead to developing Type II Diabetes and the many health risks associated with it. Your PCOS diet should involve eating foods that release the energy slowly, and these will often be referred to as Low-GI or Low-GL foods.

Your diet should put an emphasis on eating mainly organic and unprocessed foods, whenever possible. We consume toxins everyday in our foods and, especially with PCOS, it's important to try to avoid anything that will upset the natural balance of your body further and prevent your body working efficiently.

Any diet for PCOS should mention exercise, even if it doesn't include an exercise program. A mixture of cardio and lean muscle-building exercise will give an important boost to your body's metabolism and generally improve your mood and wellbeing.

Finally, there are a number of vitamins and minerals that benefit women with PCOS and any diet should offer advice on the main ones you need to be getting, either naturally in your food or as supplements.

When you are looking for PCOS diets the most important thing to avoid is any diet that offers instant or lightning-quick results. Losing weight and keeping it off permanently takes time and there are no miracle cures. Remember, this is about your overall health and not just a quick fix. If you have any doubts about what you should be eating, consult your doctor or a qualified nutritionist, and then stick to the program you have chosen.

# TABLE OF CONTENT

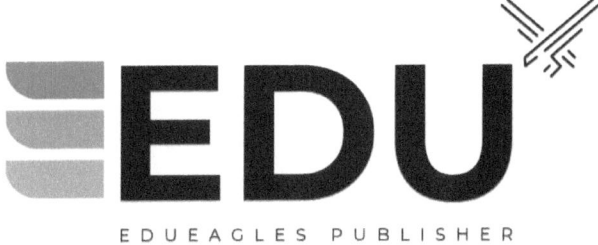
EDUEAGLES PUBLISHER

Knoledge is power

# WHAT IS A PCOS DIET?

In treatment of Poly-cystic Ovarian Syndrome the PCOS diet plays a key role but there are many diet programs out there and how you can rely upon them that these are good diets for PCOS patients. If you search for a good PCOS diet you must look that it should not eliminate necessary nutrients. A very good diet will give you a control over your weight and hormonal balance. For women PCOS can cause serious problems like infertility so must be careful about the diet and intake of other elements such as sugar and carbohydrates.

As you might know that PCOS affects almost 10 to 15% of all women. It is always a advice that your should take a healthy diet in guidance of your health professionals who may suggest some stimulants for fertility. As PCOS is left untreated it can lead to myriad problems including cancer, heart disease, and diabetes. The insulin is the main reason for fat and problems like sugar so experts suggest that a low glycol diet must be a part of treatment plan.

The cause of PCOS is still not known but from research and studies most experts believe that insulin plays a vital role. The primary problem in PCOS Syndrome is insulin resistance in that condition the insulin is not produce in adequate amount from fat, muscle and liver cells.

If you are careful to the symptoms you can better cure the PCOS some of the symptoms are indexed below:

- ✓ Depression
- ✓ Fatigue
- ✓ High blood pressure
- ✓ Weight gain
- ✓ Difficulty losing weight
- ✓ High blood sugar
- ✓ Increased blood triglyceride levels

Many researchers have found that there are special diets available that can help fighting your insulin response and weight gain. And all it takes to do is to understand carbohydrates.Mainly two types of carbohydrates are there: simple and complex. The Simple carbohydrates can be found in many processed foods such as pasta, bread and absorbed by the body very much faster than others and this causes leading sudden increase in blood sugar and so they are identified as high glycerol foods. Where as Simple carbohydrates are named as the "bad" carbohydrate and must be curbed or eliminated if you are suffering from PCOS.

The Complex carbohydrates can be found in various food items as wholegrain breads, oats, muesli, fibrous vegetables. They also contain good amount of fiber. These carbohydrates have a property of breaking down into glucose very much slowly than other simple carbohydrates so it can provide energy throughout the day. if you are having natural PCOS diet then natural complex carbohydrates are better choice for you.

As you should take low glycol food but additionally it is very much important that the intake of carbohydrates should be always with protein or good fat such as olive, canola oil or part skim cheese. To maintain the level of carbohydrate consumption you should take large amount of decaffeinated drink throughout the day because a low level of carbohydrate can lead to dehydration.

So summarizing all, a PCOS diet enriched with fiber-rich complex carbohydrates which include whole grain foods and vegetables, fruits will definitely help you to recover from PCOS syndrome and also helpful for other body related issues .

# HOW TO USE PCOS DIET

PCOS or Polycystic Ovary Syndrome is one of the common reasons why women cannot bear children. A lot of women worldwide struggle from this condition, ni fact some estimate it at 1 in 10. It is first and foremost an endocrine disorder which means it's related to abnormalities in hormones. The problem with it is its exact origin is still unknown by experts but there can be a result of a genetic disease due to a strong evidence. It's also not easy to pin point since its symptoms are a conglomeration of different conditions that are troublesome by themselves.

The most common symptoms are obesity, high cholesterol levels, and type 2 diabetes. It's most devastating effect however is the patient's inability to conceive a child. Experts however suggest that there are natural ways in order to prevent or reverse the effect of PCOS. This is through undergoing an extensive diet program to combat the multiple symptoms which characterize the condition. It would ultimately wane the overall effect of the disease itself once it is strictly followed. A lot of PCOS diet information is available for you to try out and you can find them online or on some published literature dedicated solely on the improvement of PCOS patients.

## How the diet works

The PCOS diet is concerned mainly on eliminating its obvious signs such as obesity and diabetes. The diet therefore is mostly related to alleviating both conditions altogether through eating food which can improve on the said conditions and avoid those which can worsen them. Good PCOS foods are evidently those low in sugar and cholesterol because both are respectively the main things worsening diabetes and obesity. Those foods high in sugar and cholesterol are considered bad PCOS foods. A healthy diet of food and vegetables with just the right amount of protein is therefore very helpful in alleviating the effects of the disease. The diet requires the patient to avoid sweets and food loaded with too much carbohydrates and fats.

## The role of exercise

Every PCOS diet information guide recommends proper exercise aside from just following up on the diet. Without exercise, the diet itself is relatively useless. This is because all the excess in the body can only be removed through exercise. Even

if you go on a diet you still won't lose that much fat that is already in your system. The same thing goes with your sugar levels. Physical activities will burn up sugar in our system and utilizing them as energy. Thus your sugar levels will be much easier to maintain with the proper exercise. A lot of those suffering from this dreadful condition have improved their health following that diet and exercise program meant for PCOS patients. A lot have even been able to conceive normally.

# BENEFITS OF A PCOS DIET

Losing weight and eating right with PCOS can be tough. The PCOS body doesn't process insulin normally, so a controlled diet should be adhered to remain healthy. But if weight loss isn't on your agenda, how can a person with PCOS eat right and how different is that diet than what you're already use to?

The key for PCOS sufferers is the same non-sufferers: Balance. You don't need to go out and purchase special foods that are only for PCOS sufferers. The best thing you can do is to stick to a diet of veggies, fruit, whole grains and lean meats (stay away from processed foods, this is even more important for women with PCOS). Another good tip is to start reading food labels at the grocery store, if you don't already. Try to buy foods with high fibre and avoid low fiber foods like regular pasta and white rice.

Reading food labels is just the beginning, however. You have to understand what you're reading to get the full benefit. Foods that are listed as "fat-free" sound like something you would want to add to your diet, but be careful. Most of the time, these foods are high in sugar, and that can be bad news for women with PCOS. At the same time, foods that are listed as "sugar-free" can still raise your insulin level if they contain high amounts of white baking flour or other high-carb ingredients. The best thing to do to satisfy your sweet tooth is to look for foods like sugar-free Jell-O, diet pop, Crystal Light and sugar-free popsicles because they are not only sugar free, but carb free, as well.

If you can't stay away from those refined carbs, try to slow them down by adding protein or a little fat. If you have to have bread with dinner, try putting some peanut butter or, even better, hummus on it. The addition of the protein or fat will slow the absorption of the carbs into your blood stream and help keep the insulin levels down, too.

Also, don't forget that not all fats are created equal. Try to stick with the healthy fats found in foods like nuts, avocados, fish, canola and olive oil, as opposed to foods high in saturated fats such as margarine, cheese, red meat and mayonnaise.

Finally, some common sense tips to keep in mind when it comes to eating right with PCOS. The most important thing is attitude. Don't get down about not having your favourites and stay positive about what you can have. You will feel better, look better and be happier if you don't look at your PCOS diet as a burden, but as a chance to try new things and feel healthier.

Try not to get frustrated because you don't lose weight right away, the goal isn't necessarily to shed pounds quickly, a healthy diet is a long-term eating plan to keep your body healthy. Lastly, please consult a doctor before you make any drastic changes to your eating habits or patterns. You should already have a doctor helping you with your PCOS, have him or her recommend a dietician who can help put together a diet that will work for you!

## PCOS DIET
## RECOMMENDATIONS

Not many know it, but some medical experts say the root cause of PCOS is insulin resistance. Insulin resistance is the inability of insulin to function normally and control blood sugar levels in your body. Since 80% of PCOS sufferers have insulin resistance, it makes sense for you to get good PCOS diet recommendations that focus on foods to correct insulin resistance.

First, you can correct insulin resistance by lowering your intake of carbohydrates. I recommend you start eating foods with a low Glycemic Index (GI) rating. In case you didn't know, the Glycemic Index is a rating scale that compares how carbohydrates affect your blood sugar.

Foods with a low GI score, such as proteins, whole grains and green vegetables cause a slower rise in your blood sugar. So choosing foods with a low GI rating is critical when you are suffering from PCOS because they help prevent your blood sugar level from spiking or rising too fast. It's important to know that carbohydrates tend to cause a rapid increase in your blood sugar.

Second, start adding more protein to your diet. Foods that are high in protein help control the absorption of carbohydrates. This, in turn, helps keep your blood sugar in check. Good protein choices include: lean beef, fish, chicken and turkey breast, whole eggs, beans, nuts, seeds, soy milk and green vegetables. By combining carbohydrates with proteins helps your insulin levels stay low by slowing the rise of sugar in your blood. So, for example, don't just eat toast for breakfast. Add a protein food, such as an egg. Or instead of eating just an apple, add some peanut butter.

Third, make sure you're eating plenty of healthy "good" fats and oils. And cut down on unhealthy "bad" fats. Start using Omega-3 and Omega-6 oils such as olive oil, coconut oil or canola oil. These good fats and oils are especially important for keeping your insulin levels in balance. Some of the best foods recommended for increasing the healthy fats in your diet are: oily fish, like salmon, tuna and sardines; nuts and seeds, like almonds, walnuts and sunflower seed; and avocados. So whip up some fresh guacamole dip and enjoy!

Fourth, take your vitamins, especially B Vitamins. The B vitamins are critical for helping ease the symptoms of PCOS. Here is the reason why: Vitamin B2 helps to turn fat, sugar, and protein into energy and Vitamin B6 is critical for maintaining hormone balance. Start taking a high quality vitamin B-Complex every day, starting today.

Fifth, spice up your food and drinks with cinnamon. Did you know cinnamon is rapidly becoming well-known for its ability to keep your blood sugar even and steady. In fact, it's highly recommended for people with diabetes, which is a condition related to improper functioning of insulin and blood sugar. Taking cinnamon will definitely help get your blood sugar and insulin levels under control.

Finally, I know it's important for you to

get valuable recommendations for a PCOS diet that is simple and easy to follow. More important, you need reliable diet recommendations that tell you the right foods to eat to help lower your insulin levels, decrease your blood sugar and relieve the symptoms of PCOS.

Most important of all, the best PCOS diet recommendations for you must be based on thoughtful practical information and genuine real-life solutions.

# PCOS DIET - AN EFFECTIVE SOLUTION FOR FEMALES

Many women suffer from a condition that is known as Polycystic Ovarian Syndrome. This is a very challenging medical condition that involves imbalances with the hormones. It can result in many serious health problems that could affect not only a woman's quality of life, but her life in general. Yes, that is right - PCOS is potentially life threatening. There are many different treatments available for women that experience this disorder of the reproductive system. One of the first courses of action when it comes to treating this condition is making adjustments to the diet. In this guide to optimizing the health while living with PCOS, you will be introduced to the PCOS diet.

If you suffer from Polycystic Ovarian Syndrome, it is important to understand that the PCOS diet may benefit you in many ways. Not only will it assist in alleviating the uncomfortable symptoms of the condition, but it has the potential to prevent more serious health complications from developing such as the insulin disease diabetes and the onset of heart disease. When starting any type of diet for the purpose and intent of optimizing your health, it is absolutely essential to understand that a diet is not simply changing the foods that you consume. A diet is actually a behavior modification system that will assist you in living a more productive, healthier life. Once you establish the fact that a diet involves not only changing the foods that you consume, but that it also involves changing the behaviors that you have that are associated with food, you are ready to learn how to participate in the PCOS diet.

Once you have a good and educated level of knowledge on what a diet is, you must determine how you will incorporate exercise into the diet. Regardless of what type of diet you are on, it is essential to get a fair amount of physical fitness. You must work your body in many ways. There are many physical exercises that have been proven to be highly beneficial to the female that suffers from PCOS. Examples of these exercises include walking, jogging, swimming, stretching, lifting small weights, running, hiking, bicycling, and other forms of fitness. You should work to ensure that you get anywhere from a half hour to an hour of physical exercise daily in order to ensure your success when participating in the PCOS diet. When participating in the PCOS diet, it is important to ensure that you carefully select the foods that you consume. You should work to make certain that you eliminate all processed foods in your diet and stay clear of sugars that are considered to be refined. It is important to choose foods that contain a high level of fiber. It is also important to choose only those foods that contain a high level of carbohydrates that are considered to be complex. It is also essential to ensure that you select foods that contain a lot of multi grains. It is absolutely wonderful to have a large selection of fruits and a variety of vegetables in your PCOS diet. By choosing to engage in a complete behavior modification program that involves physical activity and consuming healthy foods, you will find that you suffer less from the symptoms associated with Polycystic Ovarian Syndrome.

# PCOS DIET - IS THERE REALLY A WAY TO HELP WOMEN WITH POLYCYSTIC OVARIAN SYNDROME?

PCOS, or polycystic ovary syndrome, is a condition characterized by the development of "cysts" on either or both ovaries, resulting in irregular or absence of menstruation. These cysts are actually follicles with are fluid and hormone-filled. Normally, the ovaries produce follicles every month. One follicle is expected is mature and produce an egg, which will be released (a process called ovulation). It is ovulation which makes pregnancy possible. In PCOS, the follicles do not develop fully enough to produce and release an egg. There is also an excess of male hormones in this condition, causing excessive body and facial hair, overproduction of oil, acne, dandruff, obesity, baldness and skin thickness and discoloration. Because of the changes this condition brings about, women with this condition have to adjust their lifestyles, including shifting from their regular diet to an appropriate PCOS diet.

PCOS is also believed to be related to insulin resistance, which prevents the body from breaking down sugar. This is why diet plays a big part in lifestyle modification in women with PCOS. Here are two diet plans recommended by experts.

## Reduced Calorie Diet

Women with PCOS often experience weight issues, high cholesterol levels, and high blood pressure. Therefore, this diet addresses these concerns, with the ultimate goal of bringing down abnormally high glucose and cholesterol levels down. Small meals concentrated on biological protein, fiber, fruits and vegetables are essential. Avoid calorie-laden foods. This diet is best utilized with regular physical exercise.

## Low Glycemic Index Diet

There are two types of carbohydrates - complex and simple. Foods with simple sugars are made with refined white flour, and are digested by the body easily, resulting in a high blood sugar. Foods with simple sugars are called high glycemic food. PCOS - affected women have malfunctioning insulin systems, so complex (low glycemic) carbohydrate foods are better, since they are also usually a good source of fiber. Foods like whole grain products, fiber rich veggies and fruits help

regulate the release of sugar into the blood, to prevent an undesirable insulin reaction.

Although women with PCOS are not generally on a restricted diet, a PCOS diet should abide by the cardinals of healthy eating - high fiber, low fat and sugar, moderate protein, and good levels of vitamins.

# YOUR DIET AND PCOS - LOSE WEIGHT WITH FREE PCOS DIET PLAN

If you need PCOS help, are struggling with PCOS and losing weight, or would like to know how treating PCOS naturally can help, then you will find this following eating plan highly beneficial. PCOS is a frustrating thing to be stuck with but take heart that it can be primarily treated through fixing your diet. Use the following free PCOS eating plan as a guide:

**The Pcos Eating Plan Day 1:**

## Breakfast:

- ✓ 2 hard boiled eggs
- ✓ 1 cup melon
- ✓ 3/4 cup Whole Grain Total® cereal
- ✓ 1 cup 1% milk

- ✓ Snack:
- ✓ 1 apple
- ✓ 2 tablespoons peanut butter
- ✓ Water

## Lunch:

- ✓ 2 cups lettuce
- ✓ 1 cup other vegetables (like onions, peppers, tomatoes, carrots, and celery)
- ✓ 1/4 cup feta cheese
- ✓ 2 T Greek dressing
- ✓ 1/2 whole wheat pita Crystal Light
- ✓ Snack:
- ✓ Yogurt parfait: 8 oz light yogurt
- ✓ 1/2 cup unsweetened frozen berries
- ✓ 1/2 cup Kashi® cereal
- ✓ Diet soda

## Dinner:

- ✓ 4 oz. baked salmon
- ✓ 1 cup steamed mixed vegetables

- ✓ 3/4 cup brown rice
- ✓ 1/2 cup sugar free Jell-0® with 2 tablespoons Cool Whip®
- ✓ Flavored seltzer water
- ✓ Snack:
- ✓ 4 cups microwave popcorn
- ✓ 1 cup 1% milk

Eating a well balanced diet is the key to a healthy lifestyle for young women with PCOS. Controlling your insulin level with PCOS is absolutely essential to successfully overcoming it. Carbohydrates increases the insulin in your blood the most. You do not want this to occur.

Following and eating plan will help to control your insulin levels and ultimately rid you of PCOS. There are thousands of healthy and delicious alternatives and foods for you to choose that will change your life by minimising the impact PCOS has on it.

# THE PCOS DIET - WHAT WE KNOW ABOUT LOSING FAT AND KEEPING IT OFF FOR GOOD .

Not everyone with PCOS is obviously overweight. But the health of everyone with PCOS is threatened by the body chemistry that results from eating either a standard American-type diet, or a vegetarian diet.

PCOS is a version of what is also known as Metabolic Syndrome, or Syndrome X. This is the condition that results in men, women and sadly in recent years more and more children, when we overeat a highly processed, artificially flavored and preserved, high refined flour and simple carbohydrate diet.

The excess of sweets, breads, pastas,

cereals, and packaged foods too often provides many more calories than the average person uses in a day. Even organically grown grains, eaten whole or manufactured into 'wholesome' forms of old favorites like chips and cookies etc, will create the same problems as excess sugar, when over eaten. The insulin required to process all the blood sugar that results from a high sweet, high flour products diet, is what in turn causes higher levels of testosterone in women. This is what then leads to the hormone imbalances that cause polycystic ovaries, infertility, acne and facial hair, plus scalp hair thinning. Left unchanged, this diet will eventually cause obesity, diabetes and heart disease. It creates a higher risk for certain cancers as well.

## High carbohydrate food:

- ✓ Elevated insulin
- ✓ Elevated testosterone
- ✓ Menstrual disorders
- ✓ Facial and body hair coarsens and darkens
- ✓ Scalp hair thins
- ✓ Acne
- ✓ Increased risk for infertility, obesity, diabetes heart disease and certain cancers

Vegetarian diets are by definition high in plant food carbohydrates and low in good quality protein of the sort required by the human body to function optimally. If a person eats a poor quality diet for a long time, and then switches to vegetarian diet, the increase in fresh vegetables and fruits and nuts is a smart and

healthy addition that will lead to greater

well being. However, as a long term choice, a vegetarian diet will always lead to malnutrition.

Whoever you are and whatever your weight loss needs are there are three things that will always be true:

- ✓ There is a way we eat to get fat,
- ✓ There is a way we eat to lose fat, and
- ✓ There is a third way, different from the other two, that we eat for the rest of our lives to maintain a lean, healthy body.

This last step has been a neglected and is key feature in most people's weight loss and re-gain history.

How we eat to lose weight is different from a healthy life long diet.

Transitioning to a life long healthy diet is a life long effort that asks you to learn new information, change some habits, commit to using some form of ongoing, skillful support.

Very regular exercise is an absolute requirement for restoring your good health. In order to be able to eat a satisfying and nutritious diet without gaining fat, we all have to have good muscle tone that we maintain with regular exercise. When you don't have enough muscle to use up the fuel you eat, you will store it as fat. The more muscle you have, the more you can eat to fuel your muscles, without storing fat.

As we age, our metabolic rate naturally slows down. Dieting to lose fat also slows down the rate at which we burn calories to fuel our body's activities.

Once you have extra fat, you have to eat in a special way, for what I call a 'therapeutic interval". There are certain changes you have to make and a certain amount of time is required, for fat loss to be fully successful. This special way of eating is NOT the way you will eat the rest of your life, IF you include building muscle and using your muscle, while you are losing this fat. The more muscle you have, the more you must eat to be healthy. With little muscle and not much exercise, there is not much you can eat without making fat.

A sad fact is that 90% of people who lose weight do not keep it off. Research shows us that this is because most people do not have the necessary information, and the long term support needed to complete a weight loss effort. In one study that was typical of all similar research on overweight people, we see that follow up support with a health care professional makes all the difference in long term success:

✓ Attending more than 75% of follow up support visits = 92% kept weight off.

✓ Attending 51 - 75% of follow up visits = 90% kept weight off.

✓ Attending less than 51% of follow up visits = 72% kept weight off

✓ Self monitored patients = zero kept weight off.

Staying in touch, either as part of a mutual support group with a skilled facilitator, or with an ongoing, individualized relationship with your health care provider, is essential.

## How We Eat To Lose Weight

The most reliable and straightforward way to use up stored fat is a diet that eliminates unnecessary sweets and starchy carbohydrates, and provides plenty of fresh whole vegetables, fruit, nuts, good quality oils and lean, clean animal protein.

Every successful weight loss diet is a ketogenic diet. A ketogenic diet is one in which we reduce our total calories eaten to below the amount of calories our bodies use in a day. This will always trigger the release of energy stored as fat in our body cells. This fat is in the form of chemistry called ketones, which our muscles use as fuel. Of course, there is a big difference between semi-starving yourself, and reducing your calories in a way that keeps you satisfied and healthy!

Ultimately our long term success at maintaining fat loss requires that we feel good during and after weight loss. Maintaining steady energy levels, enjoying stable moods and having the fun and excitement of creating your own desired changes is key to your successful.

It turns out that you can burn up more

fat while eating a larger number of calories when you eat fewer of your calories from carbohydrates and more from good quality protein and fat. This type of ketogenic diet does not mean over-eating huge slabs of meat. It does not mean over-indulging in fried or fatty foods or completely eliminating carbohydrates.

Some people have misused the idea of lower carbohydrate ketogenic diets, by misinterpreting the intention of the clinicians promoting this method. As a result the media and some medical authorities have seemed to emphasize the 'dangers' or failures that followed the extreme behaviors chosen by some people. In fact, overwhelmingly, the research shows that a lower carbohydrate ketogenic diet is safe and effective for fat loss.

Remember, we can only lose fat by reducing our calories from food to less than the amount of calories we use in our daily activities. This is a fundamental truth. However, there are any number of additional details that make this strategy more or less likely to succeed, especially over time. Some conditions that complicate the basic calories reduced= fat reduced equation include:

- ✓ Chronic stress that fatigues your adrenal function
- ✓ Chronic pain that keeps your nervous system on high alert
- ✓ Insomnia that reduces the opportunity for your organs to perform restorative functions that will not happen except during deep sleep
- ✓ Perimenopause or other conditions that alter your reproductive hormone functions (including the

use of contraceptive hormones, hormone replacement therapy, hysterectomy, breastfeeding for instance)
- ✓ Thyroid disorders
- ✓ Kidney disease
- ✓ Any immobilizing condition

All of these conditions can be addressed with a diet plan and a transition plan that is personalized to your situation.

One detail important to our success at weight loss has to do with how we feel - physically, mentally and emotionally- when we reduce calories. If we just eat less, without regard to the composition of our diet-that is, the fat, protein and carbohydrate content, as well as the vitamins, minerals we need - we can have a pretty unpleasant experience. Between meals hunger, fatigue, headaches, muscle spasms, mental fogginess, emotional depression or irritability and insomnia are the common experiences shared by all dieters who use low fat, low calorie, high carbohydrate diets. With these diets, we can also find ourselves losing weight that includes our muscle mass, and not just the fat we intended to lose.

A lower carbohydrate ketogenic diet, in which we reduce our calories from starchy carbohydrates in particular and nourish our selves with appropriate amounts of water, vegetables, fruit, eggs, poultry, fish, meat, nuts and good quality oils, creates fat loss without the usual unpleasant side effects. It also helps identify problem foods, so that when we transition from a fat loss to a healthy weight maintenance way of eating, we can do so without returning to old food-related problems.

# Ketosis Is Not Ketoacidosis

Ketones are a product of fat metabolism, and function as a source of energy for the body. Our muscles and other tissues can use ketones for fuel instead of glucose, or blood sugar. Ketones are released from stored fat and are used for energy when there is not enough glucose available. Your brain requires blood sugar for fuel, whereas muscle and other metabolic processes will take up ketones instead. We can make blood glucose from everything we eat, including by transforming proteins from animal foods. We can not however, make protein for our bodies from plant foods. What we make from the carbohydrates of plant food is fat. The excess carbohydrates we eat every day beyond what we use in the exercise of our muscles, is transformed to fat and stored. This is a great system for people (like our human ancestors) who do not have a reliable food supply and are subject to regular periods of feast or famine. For most of us it means an ever enlarging "storage bin" of accumulated fat.

There is some confusion regarding the ketosis that occurs when we are eating less carbohydrates than we need for daily fuel and begin to burn stored fat instead. Some people confuse normal and beneficial ketosis with another situation, called ketoacidosis. Ketoacidosis occurs when people with high levels of blood sugar (diabetics) produce high levels of ketones at the same time.

People with diabetes do not produce enough insulin from their pancreas, or have a condition called insulin resistance, in which the tissues will no longer respond to the presence of insulin bearing glucose to be delivered into storage. Ketones are formed in response to the tissues need for some fuel other than the glucose, which is collecting in the blood attached to insulin molecules but can't be delivered into cells any more. Normally our body will adjust the blood pH level to balance this shifting chemistry. In diabetics the imbalance is too great and

ketoacidosis, or increased acidity of the blood occurs. Metabolic ketoacidosis in people with diabetes is a dangerous condition and should be avoided with very strict control and attention to diet and blood sugar levels.

When a person with normal blood sugar levels is producing ketones by breaking down fat for fuel, and is not eating excess carbohydrates, the blood glucose is delivered elegantly, primarily to the brain, and the rest of the body happily uses ketones to run the show.

Eating carbohydrate foods in amounts that allow for the release of ketones from stored fat is a safe and effective way to reduce body fat while maintaining an even blood sugar levels. Stable blood sugar means you will have plenty of physical energy, mental alertness and restful sleep. Most people can eat this way for the rest of their life and be quite well, and, most people will want to diversify their diet after having lost excess fat. Expanding your diet to include more fruits and grains as well as appropriate celebratory treats, can be accomplished with out regaining fat.

This transition has to be done thoughtfully and with close attention to the impact of certain foods. Some people will not be able to eat certain foods, ever, without negative consequences, because of our genetic make up. All of us have to reintroduce foods carefully and maintain exercise levels life long, in order not to regain lost fat.

A ketogenic fat loss diet is not appropriate for pregnancy and breastfeeding. These are times when fat stores are very important to mother and baby's well being. People with kidney damage should not use this diet unless they will be closely supervised by their physician. People with diabetes, epilepsy, and gall bladder problems also need special care and support to use a ketogenic diet successfully.

Women lose weight somewhat slower than men; feminine hormones effect how women hold onto water and fat. Men in general have greater muscle mass, even when quite fat. This fact plus masculine hormones help them burn fat somewhat more effectively than women. Regular exercise is absolutely necessary for everyone's long term health.

How we transition from fat loss to long term healthy diet determines our long term success.

Transitioning successfully from a fat loss diet to a healthy life long diet is only beginning to be understood. Specifics for success include:

- ✓ A metabolic readjustment period (5 to 10 or more weeks), and
- ✓ Educational support that works with the habits of thought and feelings surrounding body image and our learned eating and exercise behaviors.

Whenever we let go of stored energy (aka fat) by reducing our caloric intake, primitive protective mechanisms in our brains kick in. Our basic metabolic rate starts to slow down. We actually start using less fat to protect us from what our ancient brain thinks is a famine. For the original humans, an unreliable food supply made this trait essential for survival. For those of us who are eating less by choice, this mechanism is what will cause us to regain weight we have lost as soon as we start eating 'normally'" again.

That 'normal' eating concept is key. If you get fat, then eat to lose fat, and when you have reached your goal weight, you resume eating the way you did that got you fat in the first place... well, there you have it. Not only are you eating fat-making food again, you are piling this into a body that is programmed to burn less energy doing your regular daily activities. You have also have lost muscle mass To complete the change to a forever-leaner you, losing the fat is only

Step One.

Step Two is working to reset your metabolic rate to where is was or higher than it was, when you were fat. How that is done has been a mystery that frustrated the vast majority of dieters and caused a great deal of unhealthy and frustrating yo-yo patterns of weight loss and regain.

Remember that we know that 90% of people who lose weight regain what they lost, plus more. Some people do not regain however and recent research has examined what is different about this fascinating 10%. In a nutshell, what these folks do differently is to be acutely aware of small amounts weight regained, and they return to their weight loss behaviors for brief periods of time to correct the small regains. Eventually, as long as they maintain essentially healthy habits, including their food choices and exercise levels, the episodes of regain stop and they stabilize at their new weight.

Transitioning to healthy eating after losing weight requires:

- ✓ You arrive at you goal weight having established a regular, fun exercise habit
- ✓ You keep very close tabs on your weight and on your inches at waist and hips, and
- ✓ You return to weight loss behaviors whenever you have regained 2 to 3 pounds.
- ✓ You make this return to weight loss behavior then expanding out you food choices again and again until eventually you have stabilized at you goal weight with your new commitment to and enjoyment of regular exercise.

✓ You continue to maintain a healthy muscle mass, activity level and always adjusting diet of fresh whole foods as you age and/or encounter new circumstances or health challenges .

Remember there is one way we need to eat to lose fat, and then another, more generous and complex way we can eat once our goal is attained. The nature of the transition between these two ways of eating is essential to long term success. The ability to lose weight, change the diet to a less stringent, more varied one and return as often as needed to the weight loss regime for brief periods until stabilized, is apparently a rare ability. Most people do not seem to discover this behavior spontaneously. Thus long term guiding support seems crucial.

A number of studies on successful weight loss have clarified that knowledgeable support helps people remember not only the basic straightforward steps of the diet cha-cha, but also expands your skills for stress management, your exercise options and your cooking skills. Often you whole family benefits from what you have learned and how you alter your own habits.

We have many behaviors and beliefs that affect our sense of self and our ability to pursue loving self discipline over a long term. It is clear that ongoing and specific support, in the form of an individual counseling relationship or a similar support group experience, makes success much more likely. We encourage you to use both the weight loss and maintenance aspects of the program described here, and to make it all the more likely to be useful to you by adding in regular exercise as well as regular contact with a knowledgeable and skilled support system.

# PCOS DIET TIPS WHEN EATING OUT

Not paying attention to what you are consuming when you eat away from home can ruin all of your good intentions and hard work with weight loss, particularly for those with Polycystic Ovarian Syndrome (PCOS). You have got to control your blood sugar, because if you don't, then you will not have success with losing or keeping the weight off. Taking charge is really important and being consistent with what you eat when you go out is crucial.

It is one thing when you are cooking your own food because you know what you are putting into it, but when you are not in control of what you are putting into your meals, it is very important for you to know what is going into your mouth.

It is okay, and often necessary, to ask how food is prepared so that you can stay on the path to success. If you don't do it you won't know. It is really a great idea always to ask questions about how food is prepared if you are at all unsure. A common example might be some appetizers that come with sauces. You might want to ask what is in the sauce. Some sauces are very low calorie while other sauces are super high in calories.

If you aren't aware of the ingredients you might walk out of a restaurant having consumed an incredible amount of calories, sometimes 3,000 to 5,000 in one sitting. You can't eat that much in a day and expect to lose weight. You don't want to have what has been months of effort undone with a meal that can set you back 2 or 3 pounds. You've got to take charge here.

If something on the menu is not consistent with what you should be eating, for example they add butter or cheese on top that you don't need, then ask them to leave it off. You really do have to be insistent and make sure that the food that you are eating is in accordance with what you need for you PCOS weight loss success.

In a restaurant, they are there to serve you and to meet your needs, and if what they have produced is inadequate you need to send it back. It isn't bad manners at all. Sometimes people are reluctant to send things back to the kitchen when it is not quite right, particularly if they have made already the effort to clearly communicate and express what their needs are.

Some women with PCOS related weight

problems tend to have a problem with portion control. They don't necessarily know how to put the brakes on. For portion control, the guidelines I give for most women is to look at the palm of your hand and that is about the right amount of protein to have and not more than that. Your fiber needs to be at least twice maybe 3 times as much as your protein, and your vegetable portion can be the surface area of both of your hands. It is important to not overeat if you want to have success with PCOS weight loss.

Going out to eat can be a fun way to spend time with your family and friends. Don't let worrying about food keep you from enjoying a night out, and at the same time, don't let going out to eat sabotage your weight loss progress.

# PCOS (POLYCYSTIC OVARIAN SYNDROME) WEIGHT LOSS DIET

Common symptoms of PCOS include male-pattern hair growth over the entire body, balding of the scalp, irregular menstruation, and fertility problems. Can a PCOS diet be used to minimize the symptoms of PCOS and the same time, cut unwanted body fat? The answer is yes, the PCOS diet can be used as an effective weight loss diet, and here's are the reasons why:

## 1. Fruits and vegetables rule.

The PCOS diet eliminates processed foods and other unhealthy food items from a person's daily meals. Cheat meals are generally not encouraged and, instead, PCOS patients are advised to find healthier alternatives to satisfy their cravings. Fruits and vegetables are

important for PCOS patients because these natural, whole foods help restore hormonal balance in the body.
Balancing the hormones is a tough task, but with the right diet and continuous treatment, PCOS patients experience great improvements in their symptoms in a matter of weeks.

## 2. Cutting out the sugar culprit.

Refined sugars are also not allowed in a PCOS diet. PCOS patients tend to develop insulin resistance and this condition may lead to full blown type 2 diabetes or adult onset diabetes. As you can see, PCOS affects a person's metabolism and, if it is not treated correctly, it can also affect a person's cardiovascular health.

## 3. Sensible eating is coupled with regular exercise.

A PCOS diet will not be as effective if the patient does not exert effort in getting a sufficient amount of physical activity every day. In order to stay healthy, a PCOS patient is also advised to play sports or go to the gym. The minimum required time for rigorous physical activity is twenty to thirty minutes a day. A person engaged cycling will get the same heart-healthy benefits as someone who is engaged in wall climbing. It doesn't matter what type of physical activity you choose, as long as you do it regularly, and you are consistent with your efforts.

## 4. Carbohydrates are reduced.

Too many carbohydrates in a person's diet can lead to the increased deposition of fat in the body. More body fat means your weight will be in danger of increasing an uncontrollable manner. What's interesting is that, when the body begins recovering from being overweight, the effort of losing weight becomes much easier, and will feel more natural as time goes by. This is the body's way of rewarding a person's efforts to be healthier and fitter.

## 5. Going organic.

As much as possible, PCOS patients are also advised to reach for certified organic produce whenever possible. This is done to reduce the patient's exposure to preservatives and other unnatural ingredients that are commonly present in food products that are not organically produced.

Food preservatives can negatively impact a person's natural hormonal balance, so PCOS patients have to invest in better food if they want to manage their condition well.

# HEALING PCOS WITH YOUR DIET

No matter what anyone tells you, diet is a big part of a successful PCOS treatment. The key is to eat unprocessed and whole foods which do not cause your insulin levels to spike or remain high. This will help taper back PCOS related issues like obesity, hirutism, acne and a number of other things. The ideal PCOS diet is as follows.

## Low Glycemic

Foods low on the glycemic index cause a slow and steady rise in insulin levels, if any at all. Refines, sugary and carb-laden foods cause your insulin levels to spike and should be avoided at all costs. This includes sodas, snack foods, candy, white breads and starches.

## Alkaline

Keeping an optimal PH level in your body can greatly improve your PCOS. The idea behind eating alkaline is that certain foods have an acidic effect on our body and others have an alkaline effect. In order to keep a healthy PH balance in our bodies we should consume 80% alkaline foods and 20% acidic. The typical American diet is highly acidic, which can be a breeding ground for disease, cancer and you guessed it cysts.

## Gluten Free

There are an increasing amount of studies that link gluten intolerance to PCOS. Some say that PCOS and Celiac disease go hand in hand. I can personally say that after cutting gluten out of my diet, my symptoms are 90% better.

All in all, following a diet that consists of whole, unrefined plant-based foods is the best PCOS treatment without the use of dangerous medications or other costly treatment.

# BEST NATURAL TREATMENT FOR PCOS .

Polycystic ovary syndrome, or PCOS for short, is one of the most depressing conditions befalling women. It has all the elements that can shatter self-esteem and dramatically reduce the quality of life at the stage where it matters most. This condition affects 10% of women all over the world aging 12 to 45 years old usually.

PCOS an endocrine disorder wherein the female hormonal balance is greatly upset. Experts believe that the condition is genetic in its origin, but there are no clear conclusions as to its exact cause. One thing is sure though, the host of effects related to it is dreadful. It can cause obesity and diabetes due to insulin resistance and in the worst case it can even cause infertility.

Being subjected to such conditions early in life is simply dreadful and many of those who suffer from this can end up with chronic depression. There are available treatments however in combating the disease. All it takes is acceptance and the will to fight it. A lot of those who have undergone treatment ultimately reversed the effects of PCOS and have lived normal lives, and the good thing about treatment of PCOS is the fact that natural methods are very effective in combating it. At some point there is a need for synthetic medication no doubt about it, but in thoroughly beating the disease it takes an all-natural system to do it. This is because the best treatment for PCOS is diet and exercise.

# Know The Relationship Between PCOS And Diet

Diet is very important in reversing the effect of PCOS. A lot irregularities in the body show up when you have this condition, so it is therefore paramount that food intake should be monitored, so as not to worsen the effects - and ultimately control them.

The problem with insulin resistance for example when you have PCOS means that because of the condition, sugar is not synthesize properly and thus disrupts metabolism. The underlying result is obesity and diabetes. Therefore a low calorie and sugar diet would greatly help in alleviating further damage from these conditions. Fruits and vegetables with protein from fish and other similar sources are best for this type of diet.

# The Role Of Exercise

Treatment for PCOS should involve not only diet but also a good deal of exercise. Exercise does a lot of good to the body in strengthening it and maintaining weight. In the case of those suffering from PCOS, diet greatly helps in the aspect of curbing the effects of insulin resistance. It's not easy for someone suffering from PCOS to get rid of excess fat since the condition stacks it up in the body. this is where exercise is all the more important in order to burn as much calorie so as not to store it up as fat in the body. The same thing goes with sugar levels. Exercising burns up sugar for the needed energy thus also lessening sugar accumulation .

## POLYCYSTIC OVARIAN SYNDROME DIET - WHAT WORKS .

PCOS, or polycystic ovarian syndrome, causes formation of cysts along the ovaries due to a hormonal disorder. While certain factors seem to assist in its development, such as an excess of insulin (another hormone), the exact cause is unknown. Insulin assists the body in using glucose for energy and can also store the glucose in fat for later use. Because of this, some experts believe that eating a particular diet might help PCOS symptoms improve, especially if the diet manipulates carbohydrate intake in some way. Carbohydrates are used in the body primarily as glucose.

Many diets today list carbohydrates as

either "good" or "bad" and help you make the distinction by long lists of foods to avoid or eat in abundance. Wouldn't it be easier to eat a natural polycystic ovarian syndrome diet? By this we mean not cutting out certain foods or following fad diets.

A good PCOS diet plan has several features that make it work. First off, start by realizing that all foods are needed as part of a healthy diet. Does that mean you can go wild on carbohydrates? No. But you should enjoy them in moderation as part of an overall meal plan.

Work on enjoying carbohydrates higher in fiber, which helps slow down the release of the glucose stored in the food. It makes the food last longer in your body and reduces the amount of insulin produced. Find the fiber content on the food label and shoot for foods with 4 or more grams per serving.

Second, aim for healthy lean protein. Cut out fatty cuts of meat and ground beef if you are able. Ground chuck or ground sirloin are much healthier and provide a good balance to your newfound high fiber intake. Try new ideas with beans, legumes, eggs and soy! All are great sources of protein. Protein helps keep you balanced and your energy levels high. Eat moderate amounts of lean protein at each meal and you will also feel full longer.

Third, watch the fats. Try to use omega-3 or omega-6 fats such as olive oil or canola oil. Enjoy nuts and seeds a few times a week for a healthy heart but keep the portions under control. Fat is fat whether it is heart healthy or not! It can still pack on the pounds.

# HOW TO DO A PCOS DIET CORRECTLY – THE 13 THINGS YOU NEED TO KNOW

With medical science and the internet being what they are today, you'd think it'd be easy to find out what the best diet for PCOS is. But when I first looked for answers all those years back, I found so much conflicting information that it became completely overwhelming. It was worse than the time I googled "what should I buy my mother in-law for Christmas".

Should I be eating a plant based diet, or am I supposed to go keto? But how can a ketogenic diet be better when everyone tells me I need to avoid fat? And how the heck am I supposed to "just lose weight" when every diet I've tried in the past eventually made me heavier?

After years of research and having to learn everything the hard way, the goal of this article is to make the process as easy and simple as possible for you.

The following 13 steps are the governing principles that helped me beat PCOS and fall pregnant naturally. They come from a critical review of the scientific literature, and are supported by the real life experiences of the tens of thousands of women that have taken part in my free 30 Day PCOS Diet Challenge.

If you're looking for evidence based answers to what you should be eating, then look no further. This book will tell you exactly how to do a PCOS diet correctly, in 13 practical steps.

To understand how these 13 food principles work, there are just two things you need to know about PCOS.

PCOS DietWhile medical journals routinely state that the exact cause of PCOS is yet to be identified, from a practical, what-can-I-do-about-it perspective we know it's two main mechanisms: high androgen levels (testosterone being the most famous androgen), and chronic low grade inflammation.

It doesn't matter if you have lean type PCOS and you're relatively slim, or your PCOS is expressed with the more classical phenotype where you gain weight easily, these two things are responsible for all those awful symptoms we have to deal with every day.

Once you understand these two main mechanisms, the 13 steps outlined below make a lot more sense. It also becomes apparent why the same PCOS diet plan that works for women wanting to lose weight, also works just as well for someone with lean type PCOS that is struggling to fall pregnant.

Two previous participants from my free 30 Day PCOS Diet Challenge illustrate this point perfectly. While Kendall and Hanna started with vastly different health goals, these two women both achieved remarkable outcomes by following the exact same dietary principles. Kendall joined the Challenge weighing 260 lbs with a goal to lose 90 lbs. By choosing foods like those included in this PCOS Diet Cheat Sheet she was able to blast past this goal, losing 100 lbs within a few short years.

Hanna by comparison was not overly concerned about her weight when she joined my free Challenge, but couldn't fall pregnant because she never got her period. Within months of making the dietary changes described below, Hanna managed to restart her natural cycle and fell pregnant naturally. She's now a very busy mom to gorgeous little toddler.

Making dietary changes can be about as fun as having your bikini line waxed after six months in the wilderness, but if you're anything like me, then understanding the WHY behind what you're doing makes it a lot easier to get motivated.

This is a big reason why women who do my free Challenge achieve such consistently impressive results. By not just providing PCOS friendly recipes and saying "here, eat this", but instead also sharing the information behind why you'd want to make these food choices, women find the motivation to stick with the changes long term.

Fourth and finally, get that rainbow in every day. Eat different colored fruits and vegetables as much as possible. You can use fresh, frozen or canned; just remember if you use canned vegetables to rinse the vegetables well. Canned fruit should be in light syrup.

They can be healthy options for those who don't have enough fridge or freezer space or simply don't want the hassle of fruit and vegetable preparation. Fresh is still best though! Fruits and vegetables are technically carbohydrates and will raise insulin levels so be careful not to go overboard, especially on fruit.

A healthy polycystic ovary syndrome diet doesn't have to be a pain. With a few simple changes and a plan in place you could reduce symptoms, lose weight and feel great!

My intention with this article is to use the same educational approach to set you up for sustainable success. As you're about to learn, despite the epigenetic and environmental causes of this disorder, it's what you eat that drives all of your symptoms. The flip side of course is that we can turn these same mechanisms around and use better food choices to create a long-term solution.

# HOW THE RIGHT PCOS DIET PLAN CAN IMPROVE ANDROGEN LEVELS

Androgens like testosterone are the puppeteers responsible for the majority of our PCOS symptoms. The higher our androgen levels, the worse our presenting symptoms

They interact with all our other hormones to impact our fertility, to cause unfair weight gain, to promote adult acne, and to give us not enough hair in the right places, while providing extra in the wrong places. High androgen levels are pretty much the bane of our existence.

Insulin also happens to be the hormone that makes our bodies store body fat, which is why a lot of women with PCOS find it nearly impossible to lose weight, while others often accumulate excess stomach fat despite being otherwise thin.

Putting two and two together here, since our insulin levels are controlled by what we eat, if we can implement the right diet for PCOS and eat in a way that keeps our insulin levels lower, our PCOS symptoms can improve.

I've been amazed by how quickly this effect can be seen when hearing from women who do my free 30 Day PCOS Diet Challenge. It's not uncommon for people to see early results within just a few weeks of changing their diet, which is pretty remarkable.

While quick results are always welcome, what's even more impressive is the long-term benefits of a PCOS diet. After suffering for four years with infertility, Jamie Bietzell joined my free Challenge in November of 2017.

She started applying the food principles I describe below and by January of 2018 she was getting a regular cycle for the first time in years. By April she had lost 50 pounds, by June she was pregnant, and by December she was a mom. What's more Jamie did this all without nutritional supplements or any medications. Just herself, this diet, and a lot of determination.

## Inflammation And The Best Diet For Pcos

While I might get lucky once in a while, it's pretty safe to say that most people who find my blog aren't that interested in biochemistry. But it's still very important especially if you want to understand how food affects PCOS.

In the hopes of finding a happy medium, here's the less boring, simplified explanation of the PCOS-inflammation connection:

Chronic low-grade inflammation is an inherent part of a PCOS diagnosis which means our immune systems are constantly on amber alert. Together with high androgen levels, insulin resistance, and poor diet, low-grade inflammation is viewed as a key component of the "deadly quartet" of metabolic risk factors associated with PCOS). While inflammation is good if you happen to be injured, when it happens all the time it leads to many of the serious long term health risks that are associated with PCOS. Things we don't want to think about normally like heart disease, liver disease and cancer etc..

At a more everyday level, inflammation makes a major contribution to many of the daily health issues so common amongst our PCOS community. Things like bloating, sinus congestion, low energy, brain fog, sore joints, insomnia, anxiety and depression.

Given this unfortunate starting point, it makes perfect sense that when choosing what to eat, women with PCOS need to avoid pro-inflammatory foods, and eat more of the things that are rich in natural antioxidants instead.

As you'll see throughout the 13 steps below, managing insulin levels and avoiding inflammatory foods are the two foundational ideas behind each of these principles.

## 1. Avoid Fad Diets

Almost without exception, all of the success stories from my free 30 Day PCOS Diet Challenge come from women that have tried a lot of other diets before finally discovering that a PCOS diet is a unique beast.

While we can draw on the healthy influences of the Mediterranean Diet, Whole30, and Paleo recipes, none of these are perfectly synonymous with the type of diet that works best for PCOS.

## Restriction Diets Don't Work For Pcos

The most important misconception I want you to forget is this seemingly universal belief that you need to restrict your calories if you want to lose weight.

It's simply not true for women with PCOS and avoiding restriction diets is both one of the most effective, yet radical elements of a sustainable PCOS friendly diet. If you understand that body fat accumulates because of poor insulin regulation and NOT because of excess energy in your diet, then it should be pretty obvious that restriction dieting is a fool's errand.

Since PCOS is the cause of weight gain, reducing your calories is a bit like putting your dirty socks in the dishwasher. You're simply using the wrong tool for the job. Anyone who tells you otherwise is not keeping up with our current understanding of how PCOS works.

My biggest problem with restriction dieting though is the fact that they've been shown not to work time and time again, yet they continue to be the only way we're told we can lose weight.

The most famous study showing the ineffectiveness of restriction diets reviewed 31 long term weight loss studies and found that between one to two thirds of dieters regained more weight after they finished their diet than what they lost while on it. Based on the hundreds of people I hear from at the start of my free 30 Day PCOS Diet Challenge, I'd say the percentage is closer to 99%!

So I'll say it again: The best diet for PCOS does not require caloric restriction. Traditional dieting techniques don't work over the long term.

## Why I Don't Recommend A Ketogenic Diet For Women With Pcos

While it'd be unfair to call it a "fad," the ketogenic diet seems to be a popular diet for women with PCOS that I don't think is optimal. This approach can certainly be effective, but I don't think it's the best diet for PCOS.

PCOS DietKetogenic diets require that you consume very small amounts of carbohydrates like 20 grams per day small. When you do this for several days, there's not enough glucose in your system to keep you functioning so your metabolism switches to consuming fats instead. This metabolic state mimics starvation and is known as ketosis.

Going into ketosis is a pretty amazing way to lose a lot of weight quickly, and this type of diet has been widely proven as an effective PCOS therapy. These health benefits, however, are largely a result of improvements in insulin regulation, and these same benefits can be achieved without "going keto" as I'll talk about more in Step 5.

If the keto diet is something that's piqued your curiosity before then this article on the keto diet for PCOS may be of interest. While you can find a lot of people promoting the ketogenic diet for women with PCOS, in this blog post you'll find a counter-narrative where I describe five reasons why I'm not a fan of this approach.

## Why I Don't Recommend A Plant Based Diet For Women With Pcos

I also get a lot of questions from the women who do my free 30 Day PCOS Diet Challenge asking if a plant based diet is best for PCOS. This is another legitimate approach that can certainly be effective, but after spending a lot of time looking into it further, I now think that vegetarianism is far less than optimal for women with PCOS.

I totally appreciate the appeal of a plant based diet from an ethical stand point. I used to be a vegetarian for this very reason which made it harder to accept that the best diet for PCOS includes eating animal protein.

So it's in spite of my personal bias towards the wellbeing of animals that I reluctantly acknowledge these three important facts:

Eating fish, meat, and eggs is a guaranteed way to ensure you're getting adequate amounts of all nine essential amino acids. Sure you can do this by eating a wide range of different plant based foods every day, but you need to be exceptionally skilled at it to avoid an amino acid inadequacy while also keeping your carb intake low (see Step 5 below). Of the many vegetarians I know personally, none of them seem to succeed at this.

Animal sources of protein are all highly bioavailable and the same can't be said for most plant derived alternatives. It's one thing for a food to contain an essential amino acid, it's quite another for that molecule to be readily absorbed and used in your body. Pea protein isolate may be a rare exception here.

There's some micro nutrients you just can't get in adequate amounts from a plant based diet. The most obvious example is vitamin B12, with even the Vegan Society recommending their members either take B12 supplements or consume

B12 fortified foods instead. There are many other compelling examples of this such as the powerful antioxidant carnosine and the equally anti-inflammatory omega 3 fatty acids DHA and EPA. Studies have also implied that that a creatine deficiency in vegetarians may adversely affect memory and intelligence and athletic performance

To be fair to all the women with PCOS that have achieved great results when switching to a plant based diet, I'm not saying it can't be done. It's just that it's not optimal.

I've heard plenty of success stories from women who've switch to a plant based diet and I think a lot of this has to do with the fact that they're swapping out pro-inflammatory processed foods for healthy whole foods. This is great as it's exactly what Step 2 is all about. It's just that a plant based diet is even better when you also include fish, meat, and eggs while you're at it.

## 2. Swap Processed Foods For Nutrient Dense Whole Foods

Principle 2 has to be the least surprising idea here, but there's more to this general public health recommendation when it comes to PCOS.

PCOS DietThe problem with processed

foods and PCOS is threefold. The first problem is that if you're eating processed foods, you're not eating all the good things that can help heal your PCOS. And as a general rule, processed foods contain pro-inflammatory ingredients that make your symptoms worse. The worst of these are vegetable oils, which I talk about more in Step 8, and sugar which happens to be the next step in your polycystic ovarian syndrome diet induction.

There are also a bunch of compounds in processed foods that people have good reason to be concerned about. These include suspected carcinogens like chemical food coloring, potassium bromate, butylated hydroxytoluene, and its close cousin butylated hydroxyanisole

To me processed foods are things made in factories, where engineers and food scientists collaborate to produce highly marketable products that play on our evolutionary weak-points. The priorities in this process are cost and convenience rather than health and wellbeing which is kind of counterproductive to using food as medicine.

If it comes in a package and you don't recognize all of the ingredients then I'd call this a processed food.

Whole foods by comparison, like the ones included in this comprehensive PCOS Diet Cheat Sheet, are foods your granny and great granny would recognize so these should be easy to identify.

## 3. Exclude Sugar From Your Polycystic Ovary Syndrome Diet

At the risk of becoming your least favorite person, the reality of polycystic ovarian syndrome is that quitting sugar is the most powerful step you can take to overcome your diagnosis.

When I first learned this, I freaked out. If there were sugar eating Olympics, I'd have taken the podium every year. If you've ever seen the Coney Island hot dog eating contest, that's how I used to plough through Reece's peanut butter cups and ice cream okay maybe that's a slight exaggeration but the point is I get-it if you think this sounds ghastly or impossible.

But there's just nothing good that can be said about sugar when it comes to PCOS. It causes your body to store rather than burn fat, promotes unwanted facial hair, acne, and male-pattern baldness, and it makes you feel like crap emotionally.

If you're trying to get pregnant, sugar consumption is really working against you as it's known to adversely affect egg quality, increase miscarriage rates, and reduce libido.

It would be completely naive to presume that knowing something is bad for us is enough to stop us eating it. After the long struggle I fought to break my own sugar addiction I'd never make this mistake and I certainly could never judge anyone for finding this step the hardest.

Research has clearly demonstrated a number of similarities between food addiction and drug use disorders with the latest reviews finding strong evidence of sugar addiction at a clinical level (Wiss et al. 201849). Other studies have found sugar to be more addictive than cocaine at least in rats anyway. I guess that having study participants ingest pure sugar for the sake of science would never make it past the ethics review board

Responding to the social, psychological,

and biological challenges of quitting sugar really was a key driver for me when I developed my free 30 Day PCOS Diet Challenge. During this immersive experience I seek to nourish and satisfy any potential cravings, ensuring participants are well supported during the first few weeks of this difficult step.

Karina, a previous Challenge participant, is proof that even the worst sugar addicts among us can be saved. When she started my free Challenge, Karina was so hooked on sugary foods that not only was she suffering from many of the typical PCOS symptoms, but it was making her feel like a monster around the house too. With the wellbeing of her family in mind she took the plunge and went sugar free. While there's no doubt that she struggled through this process, she stuck with it and was able to lose over 60 pounds to reach her goal weight. .

What's even cooler about Karina's experience, is that after "getting clean" she now no longer thinks about sweets anymore because she no longer gets cravings. What this shows us is that even if you're a raving sugar addict to start with, cravings are a short-term problem that go away over time. Another nice benefit of getting off sugar is that your taste buds become much more sensitive, which makes everything else taste sweeter.

While I could literally write about this all day (if only someone else would do the housework), the take home point I want you to think about is this: If you really want to beat PCOS and overcome your symptoms then you're going to need to make a choice between your long term health goals and your relationship with sugar.

## 4. Be Smart About Fruit In Your Pcos Diet

But what about fruit I hear you ask? A very good question

I've always felt close to my primate roots, because besides the Lucky Charms and ice cream, I used to eat as much fruit as your average Orangutan the sweeter the better of course.

I realized after switching to a PCOS friendly diet that fruit can be a tricky food to navigate. While it contains plenty of fructose sugar suggesting that it's best avoided, fruit can also be rich in both phytonutrients and fiber.

Here's where I landed on this one: As a general rule, fructose consumption tends to make your PCOS symptoms worse, which is why Step 3 is so important. For example, a comprehensive analysis has shown that even in people without diabetic-like health concerns, fructose promotes insulin resistance in the liver While poor liver health by itself is a common concern for women with PCOS the inflammation caused by fructose consumption can result in a long list of health problems that includes weight gain, infertility, hirsutism, gut issues, anxiety, and depression.

The presence of fiber and other nutrients in fruit appears to offset the damage caused by this sugar. Even in people with type II diabetes, the fructose found in fruit doesn't appear to adversely affect liver health (Weber et al. 201856). The upshot of all this is that whole fruit is still healthy for women with PCOS, but it pays to be smart about how you include it in your diet if you want to optimize your health outcomes.

I recommend only having whole fresh fruit and avoiding ALL fruit juices, canned fruit, or processed fruit concentrates. Also make sure to choose fruits that lean towards a tart taste and avoid those that are super sweet.

You can find a comprehensive list of common lower sugar fruits in this Beat PCOS Diet Cheat Sheet.

While you can find published data sources for the fructose content of most fruit, the natural variation found between different species as well as how ripe the fruit is when you eat it means that the best way to tell is by using your taste buds. The sweeter the taste, the higher the sugar content. This means more currants, berries and melons, and less apples, grapes, and bananas.

Most importantly I suggest limiting your fruit intake to 1-2 servings per day and by "serving" I mean approximately 1 cup, or one medium sized piece.

## 5. Eat Low Carb, & Slow Carb, From Whole Food Sources

While unlikely to take off as the next sexy diet fad anytime soon, the principles of low carb, slow carb, from whole food sources describes many of the important nuances of how best to eat carbs when you have PCOS.

In the recipes I prescribe during my free 30 Day PCOS Diet Challenge and in my free 3 Day PCOS Meal Plan I aim to achieve around 20-30% of energy intake from carbohydrates. This is "low" compared to the ill-advised amounts recommended by the USDA, but is greater than that recommended for "very low carbohydrate" ketogenic diets.

Here's why I think "low carb" is the

sweet spot for women with PCOS:

Keeping carbohydrate intake "low" reduces the amount of insulin our bodies need to produce. Since elevated insulin levels are a major driving force for almost ALL PCOS symptoms (even in women with lean type PCOS) this one's a bit of a no-brainer right?

While there's little question that ketogenic diets can be highly effective in the short term, I've yet to meet someone that has found this highly restrictive protocol a happy, healthy, and sustainable lifestyle choice. Unless you're the kind of person that has a lot of self-control and is really into food and cooking, it's incredibly challenging to eat healthily while in a truly ketogenic state (see Step 1 for more details).

Having a little carbohydrate in your system all the time is the best way to stave off sugar and carb cravings. As I mentioned before, quitting sugar is one of the most powerful steps for beating PCOS, yet it's incredibly difficult because it's so darn addictive. Our bodies and brains are hard-wired to run on carbs and when we take these away, you can expect a rebellion. Eating a small amount of carbohydrates with every meal is a great strategy for making this essential step easier and more sustainable long term.

Going slow carb on the other hand means choosing carbohydrate food sources that are digested slowly over time. Often referred to as "low GI", slow carbs cause your blood glucose levels to rise in a controlled manner, which means demand for insulin, whose job it is to move the glucose out of your bloodstream and into your cells, is nice and manageable.

Now I have some major issues with the use of the glycemic index, but for the purposes of choosing carbohydrate food sources it does provide some moderately useful guidance when coupled with the third part of this principle.

Whole food carbohydrates are things you can grow and then harvest without any processing. This means starchy vegetables like sweet potato, yam, taro, and squash. Beans and lentils are another great whole food carbohydrate, while suitable grains include quinoa, buckwheat, or red, black or wild rice.

To put all this into context, as a practical guideline, I generally recommend eating either 3 oz (85 g) of grains, around 5 oz (140 g) of legumes, or approximately 3 – 8 oz (85 – 230 g) of starchy vegetables (depending on how starchy the vegetable is) with every meal.

Bianca, a previous Challenge participant, embraced this dietary principle as a key part of her journey to beating PCOS. Eating low carb, and slow carb, from whole foods sources took Bianca from the brink of gastric surgery when she first joined the Challenge, to finally finding a way to control her weight naturally. While getting off metformin and losing 30 pounds was great, what I love the most about Bianca's success story is that when she was ready, she was able to conceive naturally and have a healthy happy pregnancy.

My Beat PCOS Diet Cheat Sheet, which is the accompanying download to this article, includes a comprehensive list of PCOS friendly, low GI carbohydrate foods if you want to get started on this principle right away.

## 6. The Best Diet For Pcos Includes

## Fish, Meat, & Eggs

Given what I've already said in Step 1 about plant based diets being less than optimal, there's another important reason to eat plenty of fish, meat, and eggs.

If you're the kind of person that finds it hard not to snack, then there's a good chance you're not getting enough bioavailable protein (and fat) in your diet. This is because, our hunger and fullness hormones are cued by protein but not by sugar and carbohydrates. When we eat good sources of protein we not only support our wellbeing, but we feel full for a long time afterwards.

One of my favorite demonstrations of this fact can be seen in the second week of my free 30 Day PCOS Diet Challenge, where I prescribe steak and eggs for one of the breakfast meals. Women who only days earlier had never been able to go without a sugary morning snack, rediscover a new satisfaction they haven't experienced in years.

This is one of the reasons why whole food sources of fish, meat and eggs are such powerful tools for supporting a good polycystic ovaries diet. Eating these hunger satisfying foods make it far less likely we'll want a bakery snack in-between meals.

When it comes to formulating PCOS friendly recipes, like those you'll find in my free 3 Day PCOS Meal Plan, I generally aim to include approximately 5.3 oz (150 g) of unprocessed meat, 6.3 oz (180 g) of seafood, or 2-3 eggs with every meal (weighed raw). Even breakfast where you can.

My intention is to have you achieve

around 100 grams of highly bioavailable protein consumption per day which matches your body's amino acid demands.

I also generally recommend buying the most well-raised fish, meat, and eggs, you can afford. We're using food as our medicine after all so I tend to think of it more as a medical expense, rather than as a living expense to be minimized by all means. Ethical considerations aside, "happy meat" is the healthiest meat, with plenty of studies proving this point

I'm always a little self-conscious when making this statement though as I realize that for many people food costs can be a major constraint and I don't want this to be a barrier to eating better. We can't let the perfect be the enemy of the good so to take a more balanced perspective here, you'll be far better off eating conventionally raised beef and vegetables than chowing down on a big bowl of free-range, grass fed, organic, vegan pasta.

## 7. Include Plenty Of Healthy Fats In Your Pcos Diet

Thanks to the nonsense propaganda we've been bombarded with for the past half century, eating more fat is by far the hardest thing for many women to get their heads around when switching to a PCOS friendly diet.

Through the far reaching interests of the food and agriculture lobby, we've all been exposed to the government's view that a healthy diet is a low fat diet. Despite government health guidelines appealing to "science" in support of their agenda, the real scientific community has been saying for decades that this is clearly not true.

In 2004, Dr Sylvan Lee Weinberg, MD, published a critique of the diet-heart hypothesis in the Journal of the American College of Cardiology and summed things up nicely. She concluded that, "the low-fat-high-carbohydrate diet may well have played an unintended role in the current epidemics of obesity, lipid abnormalities, type II diabetes, and metabolic syndromes." And that, "This diet can no longer be defended by appeal to the authority of prestigious medical organizations or by rejecting clinical experience and a growing medical literature"

This sentiment is widely shared by many of her equally well- informed contemporaries with nutrition researchers like Adele Hite from the University of North Carolina publishing thorough criticisms of the recommendations made by the Dietary

Guidelines for Americans Report.

Breaking free from the ingrained idea that fat makes us fat is a major milestone towards real results for women wanting to switch to a PCOS diet. For people that've been told all their lives that fatty meat and butter are "bad for them" this can prove a cognitive challenge. I still see it daily within my own extended family!

But once we punch through the fear and doubt that's been brain-washed into us, we can use these foods as a skillful means to achieve our health goals.

When I learned that wholefood sources of fat were good for me, I have to admit, I went a wee bit crazy on the butter and pork belly. I started eating enough saturated fat to give a cardiac surgeon a heart attack but I also monitored my metabolic health markers like fasting glucose, cholesterol, and triglycerides.

To my great surprise, all of them improved a lot!

Eating more fat is the other side to the low carbohydrate coin. Diet intervention studies reliably show that a decrease of dietary carbohydrates along with an increase in fat consumption promotes weight loss, testosterone reduction and improved insulin sensitivity in women with PCOS This is useful beyond just weight loss and the management of insulin resistance though, as these are the kinds of metabolic changes that can help restore ovulation, and reduce the effects of acne and hirsutism.

And while in Step 6 I talk about the benefits of protein to help satiate hunger, our fullness hormones are also perfectly designed to be triggered by fats. This is exactly why foods like coconuts, olives and avocado are so incredibly filling, making them great for staving off sugar cravings.

Previous participants from my free 30 Day PCOS Diet Challenge have seen these exact same results. Katrina for example, had gained 50 pounds since the birth of her daughter, was suffering from secondary infertility, and was upset by the fact that she could grow a full beard. Within months of making these dietary changes, which included eating a lot more fat, she'd lost 19 pounds of body fat and her unwanted hair was gone. But best of all, Katrina was able to fall pregnant naturally and had a "wonderful, energetic pregnancy" unlike her first where she suffered from gestational diabetes.

So the best diet for PCOS should include lots of fat. You don't need to worry about eating too much because your fullness hormones will stop you.

My definition of "healthy fats" are any fats that are sourced from whole foods with minimal prior processing (for a full list of healthy fats make sure to download this PCOS Diet Cheat Sheet). This includes saturated fats which despite what everyone else believes, are actually really good for you. While I know this might sound completely loopy if this is the first time you've heard it, belief in the idea that dietary cholesterol has an adverse effect on your health, puts you at odds with the growing body of evidence suggesting this outdated theory has run its course. Even as far back as 1991, one of the original proponents of the diet-heart hypothesis, described the effect of dietary cholesterol on blood cholesterol levels as "minimal"

For more information on this topic you

can read my 6 reasons to add saturated fat to your PCOS diet here.

All the meal plans in both my free 30 Day PCOS Diet Challenge and my free 3 Day PCOS Meal Plan follow this high fat diet principle.

I especially like to use a lot of coconut oil in my recipes as this healthy fat has been shown to help with fat loss particularly from around the stomach and thighs And I also include plenty of beef and butter since these fats are the richest source of conjugated linoleic acids (CLA).

If you haven't heard of CLA before, this family of fats is known to:

Be good for your arteries.

Help with glucose tolerance and insulin action Help reduce body fat

This is saying nothing for how much better everything tastes with a good serving of butter on top!

Of course all the usual, more widely accepted "healthy fats" apply too. Things like nuts, seeds, and avocado feature heavily in all my recipes with oily fish making a regular cameo also.

So if you want to beat PCOS then eat more fat. You'll be amazed at how much difference this step will make.

You won't "get fat" provided you're following the other 12 steps. And if you have some surplus body fat, then this is one of the easiest ways to lose it.

## 8. Replace Vegetable Oils With Healthy Fats

If you got the bit about inflammation being a problem for PCOS, then Step 8 is another no brainer. Vegetable oils are straight out pro-inflammatory so eliminating these from your PCOS diet is a fairly easy win.

Despite the name, vegetable oils are not really from vegetables at all, but rather are processed seed oils coming from soybeans, sunflower, corn, canola, cottonseed, and safflower etc. The reason these oils are inflammatory is because they have high ratios of omega-6 fatty acids.

They can also contain industrial trans fats as a result of how they're made, with an older study finding as much as 4.2% trans fats in consumer soybean and canola oils.

Industrial trans fats are really bad for us. They're highly toxic and are linked to heart disease, cancer, diabetes, and obesity. Trans fats are another great reason to avoid high processed foods because the FDA only requires these to be included on the nutritional facts label if there is more than 0.5 grams per serving.

This is a changing regulatory environment however, and it seems that trans fats are about to be phased out completely in the coming years. In the meantime, I recommend avoiding any food products that include "hydrogenated", or "partially hydrogenated" vegetable oils in the ingredients list as these are trans fats, just by another name.

During my free 30 Day PCOS Diet Challenge and in my free 3 Day PCOS Meal Plan I have women switch out vegetable oils for more PCOS friendly alternatives. I recommend using coconut oil, lard, or ghee for high temperature cooking (deep frying/baking); and using butter, olive oil, avocado oil, or macadamia nut oil for low temperature cooking (stir frying), or to have cold in a dressing.

## 9. Eat Foods That Cultivate Your Gut Microbiome

Understanding the influence of the gut microbiome on our health and wellbeing is by far one of the most exciting fields in medical research at the moment.

In just the last decade, studies have shown that the microbiome affects how much we eat our metabolism and even the way in which we absorb nutrients Beyond just an associative relationship, a causal link has now been established between the bacteria in our guts and insulin resistance and obesity

One of the main ways in which sugar is "bad" for us is that the fructose component of sugar changes our microbiome for the worse. This has been shown to negatively affect liver health while studies on mice suggest alterations of the microbiome may also reduce cognitive capacity.

Making positive changes to our gut flora is one of the biggest reasons why a PCOS diet works so well.

Some of the most valuable research that's been done in this space shows that women with PCOS have a lower diversity of healthy gut bacteria and that these differences matter. Rodent studies have even suggested that dysbiosis of the gut microbiome may play a causal role in PCOS and that improvements to the microbiome may be a potential treatment option. While this might sound exceptionally complicated, we also now know that if we want to make positive changes to the makeup of our microbiome we need only change the foods we eat

While quitting sugar can reduce the kinds of microbes that work against your health goals, eating both probiotic and prebiotic foods help support the good guys.

Probiotic foods contain live strains of healthy gut bacteria, while prebiotic foods contain a specific kind of soluble fiber that enables these microorganisms to thrive. It's like probiotics are the seed, while prebiotics are the water and sunshine.

During my Beat PCOS 10 Week Program I invite participants to try probiotic foods as one of their weekly challenges. I normally suggest starting with either coconut yogurt, pickles, kombucha, sauerkraut, kimchi, miso, or tempeh. These are all fantastic snacks that slide easily into a PCOS friendly diet, which is why I include them in my PCOS Diet Cheat Sheet.

Prebiotics on the other hand are something that come fairly automatically when following the best diet for PCOS. I say this because the best sources of these compounds are found in certain fruits and vegetables as I discuss in more detail below.

## 10. Eat Plenty Of Non-Starchy Vegetables With Every Meal

Before I started the health transformation that eventually led to me falling pregnant naturally despite years of failed fertility treatments, vegetables were something I knew were good for me, but rarely featured as a high priority at meal times.

I'm sure most people reading this will be

far more sensible about food than I use to be, but for the few who like me need reminding, non-starchy vegetables are an essential part of any good PCOS diet plan. While carbs, protein, and fats are the major components of any PCOS friendly meal, eating a wide range of non-starchy vegetables is also essential for good health.

Without wanting to bore you with an unnecessary rant about why vegetables are good for you, let me explain the three biggest reasons that motivated me to improve my delinquent vegetable habits.

The first reason is phytonutrients. Phytonutrients are micronutrients that can only be found in plants and science is just beginning to understand some of their amazing health promoting properties.

Let me use turmeric as an example. Many

people are aware that turmeric is anti-inflammatory, but this is because it's a rich source of the carotenoid

phytonutrient curcumin. This leads many people to take turmeric supplements. But as I explain in my Beat PCOS Supplements Guide, the low bioavailability of curcumin means that most (but not all) commercially available turmeric supplements pass straight through you. Now if you get your curcumin from eating plenty of fresh ginger, or enjoying regular curry dishes on the other hand, you're consuming this phytonutrient (as well as many others) as nature intended and a lot more of it is absorbed by your gut.

Over 25,000 phytonutrients have been discovered so far, and if you wanted to get scientific about it you could find some of these in almost every vegetable you look at. Carrots, tomato, bell peppers, spinach, kale, and broccoli. Seriously. Pick a vegetable and it's likely to be rich in some special nutrient.

But if you're like me and you just want to get on with your life knowing you're doing yourself some good, the take home point is that more vegetables means more phytonutrients, and more phytonutrients means better health all around.

The second big discovery which really changed my attitude towards vegetables was the knowledge that this is where many prebiotic foods come from. Prebiotic foods are high in certain kinds of fiber or resistant starch which provide the energy and carbon source needed for our microbiome to flourish. A diet low in these substances has been shown to reduce bacterial abundance, while a high intake of these non-digestible carbohydrates can improve their composition

While this is far from an exhaustive list, some of the vegetables that are known to be high in prebiotics include Jerusalem artichokes, garlic, onion, leek, shallots, spring onion, asparagus, beetroot, fennel bulb, green peas, snow peas, sweet corn, and savoy cabbage

The third good reason I decided to get my rabbit on, was the knowledge of how fiber affects our gut health. While we can't digest fiber it plays an important role in aiding the passage of food through our intestines.

One of the risks of eating a low carb diet that includes plenty of fish, meat, and eggs is that you can become constipated from inadequate fiber intake. The answer of course, is to make sure you're eating lots of high fiber vegetables like garlic, artichokes, Brussel sprouts, spinach, carrots, broccoli, beetroot, and cabbage.

When it comes to the question of how many vegetables is enough, all the recipes included in my free 3 Day PCOS Meal Plan and free 30 Day PCOS Diet Challenge seek to include two cups of non-starchy vegetables with every meal, with a particular focus on leafy greens.

This can be a lot more than what people are used to, but trust me when I say your body will thank you for it.

## 11. Cut Out Gluten And Dairy

Found in just about anything made from wheat, gluten is a protein that for some reason is particularly problematic for women with PCOS. Whether you're aware of the effects or not, foods containing gluten can wreak havoc on your digestive system and are a primary cause of inflammation.

As I explain in this article about how gut health and inflammation affect PCOS it's super common for women with PCOS to be intolerant to gluten without actually knowing it. The common term for this kind of intolerance is non-celiac gluten sensitivity which is a condition that can't be diagnosed by the normal celiac blood tests or even an intestinal biopsy.

Rather than messing around with costly and potentially inaccurate immunoglobulin blood tests, the best way to find out how gluten affects your health is to do your own experiment. It's really easy and it costs you nothing.

Avoid gluten for several months and see how you feel. You can download a copy of this Foods to Avoid Checklist to see many of the most common gluten containing foods. Assuming gluten is a problem for you, you'll need to clean it out of your diet entirely to let your gut heal properly. If you begin to feel better during this time like the majority of women who take this trial seriously do, then that should be your first clue.

You can then spend a day gorging yourself on all your favorite wheat laden foods and then see how you feel. If you feel like rubbish, then that's your second big clue!

I'm all about self-experimentation like this because there's nothing more motivating or compelling than seeing real results.

Nellsy Martinez is a perfect example of what can be achieved when applying this principle as part of a PCOS friendly diet. While taking part in my free 30 Day PCOS Diet Challenge, Nellsy eliminated both gluten and dairy from her diet as well as following the rest of the principles laid out in this article. Not only did she start feeling great, but she lost weight and started getting her periods again for the first time in years. After about 8 months, Nellsy managed to fall pregnant naturally with her beautiful baby, Vivianna.

The key to success is finding alternatives to bread, pasta, breakfast cereals, and other gluten containing food products, which is not as hard as it sounds with the right information and support.

In my 3 Day PCOS Meal Plan for example, I swap out pasta for zucchini noodles (zoodles), I use lettuce leaves instead of burger buns, and I suggest a flaxseed and almond meal porridge that's 100 times more PCOS friendly than any gluten filled breakfast cereal you'll find in most "health food' isles.

While possibly not quite as prevalent as gluten sensitivity, it's also really common for women with PCOS to suffer from a subclinical dairy intolerance. While lactose is often the culprit, many people don't realize that both the casein and whey proteins in dairy can also cause inflammation.

An important nuance to this PCOS diet principle is that butter and ghee are generally well tolerated (you'll see both of these dairy derived foods in the PCOS Cheat Sheet that accompanies this article). Ghee is essentially perfectly purified milk fat so it doesn't contain any lactose, whey, or casein, while butter contains less than 2% of these compounds in total. This amount is hardly worth worrying about given how healthy milk fat is (see Step 7 if this sounds like crazy-talk).

Again, I recommend a little self-experimentation here to discover your personal sensitivity to dairy.

Many women use my free 30 Day PCOS Diet Challenge as a starting point for this process as all the recipes I provide are completely gluten and dairy free (apart from butter of course).

## 12. Know Your Personal Intolerances

Since women with PCOS are so sensitive to inflammation, it's also worth going the extra mile to discover and then eliminate any other foods that trigger your immune system.

If after eliminating vegetable oils, gluten, and dairy you still have residual gut issues, it's worth considering extending your investigation to other potential subclinical food sensitivities. Common culprits include eggs, peanuts, tree nuts, fish and shellfish.

If you're especially unlucky and have a lot of persistent gut problems, there's an outside chance that you may also have sensitivities to the group of foods known as FOODMAPS (fermentable ogliosaccharides, disaccharides, monosaccharides and polyols).

FODMAPS are small carbohydrates found in many common foods including some fruit and vegetables that are otherwise perfectly healthy. FOODMAP sensitivity is synonymous with a condition rightly named irritable bowel syndrome (IBS) and you'll definitely want to see a functional medicine practitioner or naturopathic doctor to help you navigate your way through this challenging health issue. My brother has IBS, so I've seen firsthand what it takes to get on top of this.

While the cheapest and easiest way to investigate your personal food intolerances is to do a medically supervised elimination diet, there're a few lab tests out there that can make the process a lot less painful.

As a general rule food intolerance testing is of poor quality resulting in many inaccurate results as Chris Kresser explains beautifully in this podcast. The one lab that by far seems to have the best reputation amongst doctors I trust is Cyrex Laboratories. They offer a range of different panels depending on your needs, but you'll need your doctor to order the tests for you.

## 13. Reconsider Caffeine And Alcohol In Your Pcos Diet Plan

Without wanting to sound like the Food Grinch, it's fair to say that caffeine and alcohol don't mix well with a PCOS diagnosis.

I think caffeine is best avoided because it increases your stress hormones which in turn increases your insulin levels. Regular consumption can also decrease your insulin sensitivity making it more difficult to regulate your blood sugar levels across the day. Caffeine can disrupt sleep and promote anxiety while the acidity of coffee in particular can cause digestive discomfort, indigestion, heart burn and imbalances in our gut microbiome.

Alcohol on the other hand has been shown to be a particularly problematic substance for women with PCOS. We have higher rates of liver disease because of this disorder and even small amounts of alcohol consumption increase these risks

Moving away from caffeine and alcohol also makes it easier to avoid sugar and empty carbohydrates, which are often found in these drinks.

I'm not saying never, but these two particular beverage ingredients are well worth reconsidering.

To make this process possible, it's important to find suitable alternatives that meet your needs and I share several of my personal favorites in my PCOS Diet Cheat Sheet. Ground roasted cocoa in particular can totally transform your belief that you must have coffee in the mornings.

This is exactly why I created my free 30 Day PCOS Diet Challenge and if you're ready to begin, this is a great place to start. The goal of this free program is to make it both fun and easy for people like you to put these 13 food principles into practice. As well as the weekly meal plans, recipes, and shopping lists I've already mentioned, the 30 Day Challenge includes video lessons, and daily mindset exercises, all within a vibrant and supportive community environment.

I run the Challenge four times a year as a live event, but if you're feeling especially inspired and want to get started right now then I recommend downloading my 3 Day PCOS Diet Meal Plan also. This 15 page free ebook includes a collection of some of my most popular PCOS recipes with an accompanying shopping list and further information about how to use food to beat PCOS.

Here's the most important thing to keep in mind though when starting your journey towards a PCOS friendly diet:

Be realistic with your expectations.

While it drives me crazy whenever my mom says it to me, there's a lot of truth in the cliché that Rome wasn't built in a day.

Beating PCOS is not a race, and if it were, it'd only be with yourself.

To be entirely honest with you, it took me years to fully incorporate these 13 principles into my everyday life so I'm certainly not going to tell you this process is easy. Having the right information and support can definitely make it "easier", but even the best dietary changes can feel like a drag at times.

It's totally fine if it ever feels unfair. Because it freakin is!

Given my previously terrible relationship with food, I can assure you there was ample cognitive dissonance as I went about implementing a PCOS friendly diet. It's only because I know how hopeless I used to be, and all the short cuts I tried to take, that I'm 100% confident that anyone can get there eventually.

So take your time, and be good to yourself.

Be honest about your weaknesses, leaving your negative self-judgment at the door. Focus on your health goals, and set yourself up for success.

# HOW TO CHANGE YOUR DIET AND EXERCISE ROUTINE IF YOU HAVE POLYCYSTIC OVARY SYNDROME

PCOS - polycystic ovary syndrome - is one of the most common hormonal disorders for women. In fact, 5-10% of women have PCOS, although 1 in 5 may have polycystic ovaries

But when you've been diagnosed with the syndrome, no matter how severe your symptoms, from excess hair to spots, irregular or absent periods and weight gain, it can be really hard to know what to do next.

Firstly, it's important to remember that although PCOS is related to our hormone levels, and insulin production, it's not your 'fault' if you have it. The symptoms can sometimes, however, be managed and hopefully, improved through diet and exercise.

PCOS and weight loss/gain is also a bit of a catch 22 - it can be linked to insulin resistance, which can lead to weight gain, and then because excess body fat causes the body to produce even more insulin, this can make PCOS symptoms worse - creating a vicious cycle.

But information online is totally overwhelming when it comes to PCOS and lifestyle - is losing weight the answer? Should you totally ditch all foods that raise your blood sugar? Will exercise help?

If you are overweight, with a BMI of over 25, Mr John Butler, Consultant Gynaecological Surgeon at The London Clinic advises that "even a small reduction in weight can significantly improve symptoms - including a low mood or depression (which is often a symptom of PCOS)".

"Generally, you want to focus on 'being healthy' so try to consume lots of fruit and veg, avoid high GI food, take regular meals so your blood sugar levels aren't going up and down too much, try to do 30 minutes of exercise a day, and stop smoking".

"Polycystic ovarian syndrome is your body's way of saying you can't handle high sugar levels - so your diet is a chance to really change things – and this can help you in your later life, pre-menopause and before and during pregnancy. By keeping your weight stable, your pregnancy is likely to be more straightforward health wise".

Daria Tiesler, a Registered Nutritional

Therapist, Personal Trainer and Performance Coach at Ultimate Performance Mayfair, regularly trains clients with PCOS, and agrees that diet and exercise can really help with managing the condition.

Here are 7 ways she advises her clients to overhaul their lifestyle:

## 1. Focus on nutrition, not diet

Daria advises veering away from fad diets, and eating with a focus to fuelling your body, managing stress and balancing your hormones. For her clients, the key is to address insulin resistance and to reduce cortisol (stress hormone) levels by packing their diet with anti-inflammatory foods.

On her shopping list are lots of leafy green vegetables, blueberries, pineapples and a focus on whole foods and sources of protein like fish, eggs and chicken breast, and good fats like nuts and avocado.

Daria's also a big fan of spices like turmeric, cinnamon, fenugreek, and ginger, that are anti-inflammatory and believed to help with insulin resistance.

One of Daria's favourite foods for balancing hormones is Flaxseed which is rich in fibre and Omega 3s. She tells her clients to eat two tablespoons per day in on salads, or sprinkled on porridge or in smoothies.

## 2. Cut out the crap

Reducing foods in your diet that cause spikes in blood sugar is crucial to managing your PCOS. This means opting for wholegrain sources of carbohydrates over anything with a high GI.

Daria advises reducing your consumption of white pasta, white rice, and anything super-processed (including processed meats).

Daria also suggests swapping fruit drinks and smoothies for whole fruit, because they contain more fibre, which is vital for a healthy gut - "most of the ladies I train have problems with gut function", Daria says. Fruits low in fructose are best, like grapefruits, clementines, lime, lemon, raspberries, blackberries and strawberries.

## 3. Try and balance your blood sugar throughout the day

"Start with breakfast" Daria says "Don't leave home with an empty stomach and then grab a sandwich at 12. So many of my clients skip breakfast or have coffee and a croissant - and their bodies struggle to process it".

Try something like eggs, salmon and spinach, or a smoothie with vegan protein, a blend of berries, cinnamon and avocado. Just make sure whatever you're eating stabilises your blood sugar by including protein and fats as well as low GI carbs.

## 4. Don't fear fats

Many of Daria's clients with PCOS are scared of fats because they don't want to put on weight, but increasing healthy fats in your diet is a great way to keep you satiated, and can help your body absorb vitamins A, D, E, K and help with healthy female hormone levels.

Just as a reminder, healthy fats mean foods like avocado, salmon, mackerel, sardines butter, and olive oil (free range or organic if possible).

## 5. Or carbs

Reducing or " cutting" out processed and high GI carbs is beneficial for anyone with PCOS , but because everyone is different we need to personalise the amount of complex carbohydrates from fruits , vegetables and pulses - and there is no need to ditch them entirely. Those foods are a great source of phytonutrients, vitamins and minerals as well as fibre.

Daria recommends experimenting - try removing the processed carbs from your diet, while keeping whole foods, like pulses, lentils and beans in there and seeing how you feel. At the end of the day, a bit of trial and error might be needed to find what works for you.

"I try a macronutrient split of around 20

percent complex carbs, 40 percent protein and 40 percent fat for my clients" Daria says "but I switch it around and get constant feedback from them as to whether it's working or not".

## 6. Look out for 'hormonal disrupters'

In a body that's struggling to balance hormones, the last thing you need are factors in your life that cause more hormonal imbalances, like stress and lack of sleep. Daria advises avoiding 'hormonal disrupters' like plastic bottle and containers that contain BPAs, but also looking at the bigger picture of how stressed out you are day-to-day.

"Review the stress in your life - I train 8-10 girls at any one time with PCOS, and many of them are super strong on the outside, but totally stressed on the inside" Daria says.

"Make sure you are getting enough sleep, and good quality sleep, too. I also recommend journalling or breathing techniques to help with relaxation."

Daria advises avoiding stimulants, aka coffee after 2pm, and swapping it for spearmint tea and green tea. Mainly because a high caffeine intake is going to give you the energy crashes you're trying to avoid and can affect the quality of your sleep, but also because coffee removes magnesium from the body - and magnesium helps the body metabolise carbs, so is pretty vital.

## 7. Hit the weights - but don't stress your body out

Daria is a huge advocate for resistance training with weights for women with PCOS. "My first goal with my clients is to manage their insulin resistance my second is to increase their muscle mass" says Daria, "because the more muscle mass you have means you can better metabolise glucose and can handle carbs better".

Daria uses a mix of weight training with HIIT (high intensity interval training) and LISS (Low intensity steady state cardio, like walking) on her clients. But the key is to make sure whatever exercise you're doing is not too stressful on the body because over-exercising is not good for your hormonal balance, either.

Often clients will come to Daria and they have previously been doing lots and lots of cardio, along with prolonged low calorie and low fat diets, which she would change to 2-3 weight training sessions a week for around 45-60 mins, coupled with some swimming, walking or yoga.

# 13 HELPFUL TIPS HOW TO LOSE WEIGHT WITH PCOS

Polycystic ovary syndrome (PCOS) is a condition characterized by hormonal imbalances, irregular periods, and/or the development of small cysts on one or both ovaries.

This condition can impact up to 7% of adult women The hormonal imbalances, insulin resistance, and inflammation related to this condition make it difficult for women with PCOS to shed weight.

Yet, even a small weight loss of approximately 5% can improve insulin resistance, hormone levels, menstrual cycles, fertility, and overall quality of life in women with PCOS

Here are 13 helpful tips for losing weight with PCOS.

## 1. Reduce Your Carb Intake

Lowering your carb consumption may help manage PCOS due to carbs' impact on insulin levels.

Approximately 70% of women with PCOS have insulin resistance, which is when your cells stop recognizing the effects of the hormone insulin (3Trusted Source).

Insulin is necessary for blood sugar management and energy storage in your body. Research associates high levels of insulin with increased body fat and weight gain in the general population and in women with PCOS.

In one study, obese women with PCOS and insulin resistance first followed a 3-week diet of 40% carbs and 45% fat, then a 3-week diet of 60% carbs and 25% fat. Protein intake was 15% during each phase.

While blood sugar levels were similar during the two phases of the diet, insulin levels went down 30% during the lower-carb, higher-fat phase.

What's more, a low-glycemic diet may benefit women with PCOS. The glycemic index (GI) is a measurement of how quickly a particular food raises blood sugar.

In one study, women ate their normal diet for 12 weeks, followed by a low-GI diet for 12 weeks. Their measures of insulin sensitivity (how efficiently the body uses insulin) were significantly better during the low-GI phase (7Trusted Source).

Eating a low-GI, low-carb diet may reduce insulin levels in women with PCOS. In turn, this could help with weight loss.

## 2. Get Plenty of Fiber

Because fiber helps you stay full after a meal, a high-fiber diet may improve weight loss in women with PCOS.

In the United States, the Reference Daily Intake (RDI) for fiber is 14 grams per 1,000 calories or around 25 grams per day for women. However, the average daily fiber intake for U.S. women is only 15–16 grams.

In one study, higher fiber intake was linked to lower insulin resistance, total body fat, and belly fat in women with PCOS but not in women without PCOS

In another study in 57 women with this condition, higher fiber intake was associated with lower body weight

For women with PCOS, a diet high in

fiber may help reduce insulin resistance, body weight, and excess body fat.

## 3. Eat Enough Protein

Protein helps stabilize blood sugar and increases feelings of fullness after a meal.

It may also aid weight loss by reducing cravings, helping you burn more calories, and managing hunger hormones.

In one study, 57 women with PCOS were given either a high-protein diet more than 40% of calories from protein and 30% from fat or a standard diet consisting of less than 15% protein and 30% fat.

Women in the high-protein group lost an average of 9.7 pounds (4.4 kg) after 6 months significantly more than those in the control group.

If you're concerned you're not getting

enough protein, you can add it to your meals or choose high-protein snacks. Healthy, high-protein foods include eggs, nuts, dairy, meat, and seafood.

Higher protein intake may boost weight loss, especially for women with PCOS. Try adding healthy, high-protein items like eggs, nuts, and seafood to your diet.

## 4. Eat Healthy Fats

Having plenty of healthy fats in your diet may help you feel more satisfied after meals, as well as tackle weight loss and other symptoms of PCOS.

In one study in 30 women with PCOS, a low-fat diet (55% carbs, 18% protein, 27% fat) was compared to a higher-fat diet (41% carb, 19% protein, 40% fat).

After eight weeks, the higher-fat diet resulted in more fat loss including belly fat than the lower-fat diet, which also reduced lean body mass.

In fact, although fats are rich in calories, adding healthy fats to meals can expand stomach volume and reduce hunger. This may help you to eat fewer calories throughout the day

Examples of healthy fats include avocado, olive oil, coconut oil, and nut butters. Combining a healthy fat with a protein source can further increase the filling effects of meals and snacks.

Eating more healthy fats may be beneficial for women with PCOS. In studies, higher fat intake is linked to reduced hunger and a greater loss of body fat.

## 5. Eat Fermented Foods

Healthy gut bacteria may play a role in metabolism and weight maintenance.

Studies suggest that women with PCOS may have fewer healthy gut bacteria than women without this condition.

Additionally, emerging research suggests that certain probiotic strains may have positive impacts on weight loss.

As such, eating foods high in probiotics such as yogurt, kefir, sauerkraut, and other fermented foods may help increase the number of beneficial bacteria in your gut.

You can also try taking a probiotic supplement to get the same results.

Women with PCOS may have lower numbers of beneficial gut bacteria. Eating foods rich in probiotics or taking a probiotic supplement may support your gut bacteria, thus aiding weight loss.

## 6. Practice Mindful Eating

Women with PCOS have often tried many diets and are three times more likely to have eating disorders.

Mindful eating is one potential solution. It promotes an increased awareness of bodily cues, such as hunger and fullness.

Mindfulness-based approaches to food may help address problematic eating behaviors especially binge eating and emotional eating.

What's more, studies suggest that mindful eating practices may be linked to weight loss

Mindful eating helps promote awareness of internal eating cues and may promote weight loss. It may be especially helpful for women with PCOS, who are much more likely to experience eating disorders.

## 7. Limit Processed Foods and Added Sugars

Another tip to lose weight with PCOS is to cut down on your intake of certain unhealthy foods.

Processed foods and added sugars may raise blood sugar levels and increase your risk of insulin resistance, which is linked to obesity

Women with PCOS may process sugar differently than women without it.

Research shows that women with PCOS experience larger spikes in blood sugar and insulin levels after consuming the same amount of sugar as women without this condition

Studies indicate that minimally

processed, real foods not only raise blood sugar less than highly processed foods but are also more satisfying

Furthermore, experts recommend that women with PCOS limit their consumption of added sugars and refined carbs to manage symptoms and maintain a healthy body weight

Foods high in added sugar and refined carbs include cakes, cookies, candy, and fast food.

Processed foods such as refined carbs and added sugars increase blood sugar levels, which can lead to weight gain.

## 8. Reduce Inflammation

Inflammation is your body's natural response to infection or injury.

But chronic inflammation which is common in women with PCOS is linked to obesity. Sugar and processed foods may contribute to inflammation.

In one study, 16 women with PCOS who took a one-time dose of 75 grams of glucose a particular type of sugar had higher blood markers for inflammation, compared to women without this condition.

A diet like the Mediterranean diet which is high in fruits, vegetables, whole grains, olive oil, and omega-3-rich foods, such as fatty fish may protect against inflammation

Inflammation is common in women with PCOS and has been linked to obesity. Eating a diet high in whole foods especially fruits and vegetables may safeguard against inflammation.

# 9. Don't Undereat

Long-term calorie restriction may slow down your metabolism. Although calorie restriction is likely to lead to short-term weight loss, over time, the body adapts to this restriction by reducing the number of overall calories it burns, which can lead to weight regain

Eating too few calories can negatively impact hormones that control appetite as well.

For example, in one study, restrictive dieting was found to modify the hormones leptin, peptide YY, cholecystokinin, insulin, and ghrelin, which increased appetite and led to weight gain.

Instead of restricting calories, it may be best to focus on eating whole foods and cutting out unhealthy products.

For example, a study in over 600 people suggested that eating more vegetables and whole foods while reducing consumption of processed foods, refined grains, and added sugars may help promote weight loss without restricting calories.

Chronic calorie restriction may slow down your metabolism, possibly leading to weight gain. Instead of forcing yourself to eat less food, try to adopt a diet of whole, unprocessed foods to help with weight loss.

## 10. Exercise Regularly

Exercise is a well-known strategy to improve weight loss.

In a 12-week study in which 16 women did 45–60 minutes of cardio 3 times per week, those with PCOS lost 2.3% body fat, compared to 6.4% in the control group

While women with PCOS lost less fat than those without this condition, the exercise regimen did result in loss of belly fat and improvements in insulin sensitivity.

Weight training has also been shown to aid women with PCOS.

In one study, 45 women with PCOS did weight training 3 times weekly. After 4 months, they lost belly fat and gained lean body mass while reducing testosterone and blood sugar levels

Both cardio and weight-training exercises may help women with PCOS drop body fat and improve insulin sensitivity.

## 11. Get Enough Sleep

Sleep is increasingly acknowledged as

central to your health.

If you have PCOS, you may experience sleep disturbances, including excessive daytime sleepiness, sleep apnea, and insomnia.

Lack of sleep has been shown to increase the activity of hormones that drive hunger, such as ghrelin and cortisol, which may cause you to eat more throughout the day.

In fact, insufficient sleep is associated with a higher risk of being overweight or obese

A review of 18 studies found that those who slept less than 5 hours per night were significantly more likely to be obese.

Furthermore, the study demonstrated that every hour of additional sleep per night was associated with a decrease in body mass index (BMI) of 0.35 kg per square meter

Additionally, studies have linked better-quality sleep to fat loss.

In one study, healthy adults who slept less than 6 hours per night had a 12% higher risk of developing belly fat compared to those who slept 6–8 hours a night

Poor sleep is linked to obesity. Studies in healthy adults suggest that increasing your total time asleep can reduce body fat and promote weight loss.

## 12. Manage Your Stress

Because stress is a risk factor for weight gain, managing your stress can help manage your weight.

Stress increases levels of cortisol, a hormone made by your adrenal glands. Chronically high cortisol levels are linked to insulin resistance and weight gain

Chronic stress also increases your risk of developing belly fat. In turn, belly fat increases inflammation, which triggers your body to make more cortisol creating a vicious cycle

To lower cortisol levels, focus on stress management practices.

Studies note that techniques like meditation, yoga, and spending time in nature can help lower cortisol levels

High cortisol levels from chronic stress are linked to insulin resistance and belly fat. Relieving stress through yoga, meditation, and time outdoors may help lower cortisol levels.

## 13. Consider Supplements

If you have PCOS, several supplements may help manage weight and symptoms.

Myo-inositol is a supplement that may lead to weight loss in women with PCOS. Inositol is a compound related to B vitamins that helps improve insulin sensitivity. Myo-inositol is a specific form of inositol.

In a randomized study in 92 women with PCOS, half were given 4 grams of myo-inositol per day for 14 weeks. While those in the inositol group lost weight, those in the placebo group gained weight Carnitine, an amino acid found in meat, may also lead to weight loss.

In a 12-week study in 60 overweight women with PCOS, those who took 250 mg of carnitine per day lost an average of 5.9 pounds (2.7 kg), compared to a 0.2-pound (0.1-kg) gain in the placebo group

Myo-inositol and carnitine supplements may help women with PCOS lose weight and control certain symptoms

## What to eat if you have PCOS

Diet and PCOS Foods to eat Foods to avoid Other lifestyle changes When to see a doctor Outlook

Polycystic ovary syndrome is a condition that causes hormonal imbalances and problems with metabolism.

Polycystic ovary syndrome (PCOS) is a common health condition experienced by one out of 10 women of childbearing age. PCOS can also lead to other serious health challenges, such as diabetes, cardiovascular problems, depression, and increased risk of endometrial cancer.

Some research has shown that diet can help reduce the impact of PCOS. Learn more about a PCOS diet in this article.

## How does diet affect PCOS?

Vegan meal with chickpeas, quinoa,

sweet potato, avocado, lime, and high fiber vegetables and legumes for pcos diet

A diet that includes high-fiber foods may benefit people with PCOS.

Two of the primary ways that diet affects PCOS are weight management and insulin production and resistance.

However, insulin plays a significant role in PCOS, so managing insulin levels with a PCOS diet is one of the best steps people can take to manage the condition.

Many people with PCOS have insulin resistance. In fact, more than 50 percent of those with PCOS develop diabetes or pre-diabetes before the age of 40. Diabetes is directly related to how the body processes insulin.

Following a diet that meets a person's nutritional needs, maintains a healthy weight, and promotes good insulin levels can help people with PCOS feel better.

## Foods To Eat

Research has found that what people eat has a significant effect on PCOS. That said, there is currently no standard diet for PCOS.

However, there is widespread agreement about which foods are beneficial and seem to help people manage their condition, and which foods to avoid.

Three diets that may help people with PCOS manage their symptoms are:

A low glycemic index diet: The body digests foods with a low GI more slowly, meaning they do not cause insulin levels to rise as much or as quickly as other foods, such as some carbohydrates. Foods in a low GI diet include whole grains, legumes, nuts, seeds, fruits, starchy vegetables, and other unprocessed, low-carbohydrate foods.

An anti-inflammatory diet: Anti-inflammatory foods, such as berries, fatty fish, leafy greens, and extra virgin olive oil, may reduce inflammation-related symptoms, such as fatigue.

The DASH diet: Doctors often recommend the Dietary Approaches to Stop Hypertension (DASH) diet to reduce the risk or impact of heart disease. It may also help manage PCOS symptoms. A DASH diet is rich in fish, poultry, fruits, vegetables whole grain, and low-fat dairy produce. The diet discourages foods that are high in saturated fat and sugar.

A 2015 study found that obese women

who followed a specially-designed DASH diet for 8 weeks saw a reduction in insulin resistance and belly fat compared to those that did not follow the same diet.

A healthful PCOS diet can also include the following foods:

- ✓ natural, unprocessed foods
- ✓ high-fiber foods
- ✓ fatty fish, including salmon, tuna, sardines, and mackerel
- ✓ kale, spinach, and other dark, leafy greens
- ✓ dark red fruits, such as red grapes, blueberries, blackberries, and cherries
- ✓ broccoli and cauliflower
- ✓ dried beans, lentils, and other legumes
- ✓ healthful fats, such as olive oil, as well as avocados and coconuts

✓ nuts, including pine nuts, walnuts, almonds, and pistachios
✓ dark chocolate in moderation
✓ spices, such as turmeric and cinnamon

Researchers looking at a range of healthful diet plans found the following slight differences. For example:

Individuals lost more weight with a diet emphasizing mono-unsaturated fats rather than saturated fats. An example of this kind of diet is the anti-inflammatory diet, which encourages people to eat plant-based fats, such as olive and other vegetable oils.

People who followed a low-carbohydrate or a low-GI diet saw improved insulin metabolism and lower cholesterol levels. People with PCOS who followed a low-GI diet also reported a better quality of life and more regular periods.

In general, studies have found that losing weight helps women with PCOS, regardless of which specific kind of diet they follow.

## Foods To Avoid

- ✓ Soda or coke cola in glass with ice.
- ✓ People on a PCOS diet should avoid sugary beverages.

In general, people on a PCOS diet should avoid foods already widely seen as unhealthful. These include:

- ✓ Refined carbohydrates, such as mass-produced pastries and white bread.
- ✓ Fried foods, such as fast food.
- ✓ Sugary beverages, such as sodas and energy drinks.

✓ Processed meats, such as hot dogs, sausages, and luncheon meats.
✓ Solid fats, including margarine, shortening, and lard.
✓ Excess red meat, such as steaks, hamburgers, and pork.

Other lifestyle changes

Lifestyle changes can also help people with PCOS manage the condition. Research has shown that combining a PCOS diet with physical activity can lead to the following benefits:

✓ weight loss
✓ improved insulin metabolism
✓ more regular periods
✓ reduced levels of male hormones and male-pattern hair growth
✓ lower cholesterol levels

Studies have also found that behavioral strategies can help women achieve the weight management goals that, in turn, help manage PCOS symptoms. These practices include:

- ✓ goal-setting
- ✓ social support networks
- ✓ self-monitoring techniques
- ✓ caring for psychological well-being

Reducing stress through self-care practices, such as getting enough sleep, avoiding over-commitment, and making time to relax, can also help a person manage PCOS.

When to see a doctor

Common PCOS symptoms include:

- ✓ acne
- ✓ extra hair growth
- ✓ weight gain, especially around the belly
- ✓ oily skin
- ✓ irregular periods
- ✓ discomfort in the pelvic area

✓ difficulty getting pregnant

Many people who experience these symptoms may not consider them serious enough to discuss with a doctor. Many people do not seek medical help until they have trouble conceiving.

Anyone experiencing these symptoms should discuss their concerns with a doctor: the sooner they can begin a treatment plan the sooner they can feel better.

## INSULIN-RESISTANCE DIET FOR DIABETES

When it comes to preventing diabetes, your diet can make a big difference. And if you already have it, a diet change may help you manage it better.

The right mix of foods keeps your insulin and blood sugar in check. When you have insulin resistance, that balance gets out of whack. It's harder for your body to burn foods for energy. And when too much sugar builds up in your bloodstream, you may be on the path to type 2 prediabetes or diabetes.

And that might lead you to an insulin-resistance diet.

You don't need special foods for the insulin-resistance diet. In a nutshell, you'll eat less unhealthy fat, sugar, meats, and processed starches, and more vegetables, fruits, whole grains, fish, and lean poultry. But it can be hard to change habits. So keep some simple tips in mind before you start.

## Your Genes And Your Health

Precision medicine centers on two sets of facts about you: What your genes say and how your environment affects you.

Slideshow: Boost Your Energy Levels with cITP

Does your cITP have you feeling fatigued? Try these energy boosters for a little more pep in your step.

## Annual Checkups You Need

When's the last time you had your cholesterol, blood pressure, or weight checked? Learn which medical tests and screenings you should have and how often you should have them.

## Home Remedies For Sick Kids

Rest is best it helps them heal.

Adopt healthy habits. A crash diet won't help you. This is about changing your approach to food. Go slowly and build new habits that can become permanent. Maybe you can drink less sugary sodas. Or quit altogether.

Make it work for you. You may enjoy different foods than what others like to eat. A diet needs to fit your taste buds and your lifestyle for you to stick with it. Most people need support along the way, so a good dietitian can be a big ally.

Don't skip meals. You might think missing a meal means fewer calories and more weight loss. That just makes your insulin and blood sugar levels swing up and down. And that can lead to more belly fat, which makes your body more likely to resist insulin.

Focus on calories and quality. The debate over the best mix of carbs, proteins, and fats has no clear answers. Your best bet is to watch your total calories and to really make them count. So skip the white rice and go whole grain instead.

Mix it up. There's no magic food that'll fix everything, so vary what you eat. When you have a choice, choose the food with more vitamins, minerals, and fiber.

## What To Eat

When you fix meals and snacks, here's what to aim for.

Tons of vegetables. It's hard to go wrong here. Take dark green, leafy veggies like spinach. They're low in carbs and calories, and they're packed with nutrients, so you can eat as much as you want.

Fresh vegetables are best. If you go frozen or canned, make sure there's no added fat, salt, or sugar.

Watch out for starchy vegetables, like potatoes, peas, and corn. They have more carbs, so treat them more like grains, and don't overdo it.

Plenty of fruit. Packed with vitamins, minerals, and fiber, they're another great choice. Swap a fruit for sweets to tame your cravings. Add berries to plain, non-fat yogurt to make it into a dessert.

Again, fresh is best. Make sure to avoid canned fruits with syrup added. And remember that fruits count as carbs.

High fiber. When you eat more than 50 grams of fiber a day, it helps balance your blood sugar. Almonds, black beans, broccoli, lentils, and oatmeal and are all rich in fiber.

Limited carbs. You can eat carbs, but cut back on them and pick wisely. Go for carbs in fruits, veggies, whole grains, beans, and low-fat dairy instead of processed foods like white bread and pasta.

Whole grains that haven't been turned into flour are even better. So for breakfast, choose oats over toast.

Lean protein. You want to make sure to get enough protein, but not when it's loaded with fat. Limit beef, lamb, and pork, and stick with:

- ✓ Chicken or turkey without the skin
- ✓ Fish, such as albacore tuna, sardines, and salmon
- ✓ Low-fat cheese and egg whites
- ✓ Proteins from plants, like beans, lentils, and nut butters

## Healthy Fats.

Swapping out saturated and trans fats for healthy ones can lower insulin resistance. That means less meat, full-fat dairy, and butter, and more olive, sunflower, and sesame oils.

Low-fat dairy. With low-fat milk and plain, nonfat yogurt, you get calcium, protein, and fewer calories. Plus, several studies show that low-fat dairy lowers insulin resistance.

If you're used to full-fat, you can dial it down slowly. So maybe try 1% or 2% milk for a while before switching to skim.

## What To Limit Or Avoid

Try your best to stay away from:

Processed foods, which often have added sugar, fat, and salt. If it comes in cans, boxes, wrappers, and other packaging, it's probably processed.

Saturated and trans fats, which can boost insulin resistance. These come mainly from animal sources, such as meats and cheese, as well as foods fried in partially hydrogenated oils.

Sweetened drinks, like soda, fruit drinks, iced teas, and vitamin water, which can make you gain weight.

# WEIGHT-LOSS BREAKTHROUGH AND SHOPPING LIST .

weight-loss breakthrough relies on efficient meal prep for three weeks of better eating. Here's what you need to stock up on to make all of the recipes.

## Prep Day

From week to week, you'll have leftovers from your Prep Day: The salmon and chicken recipes, for example, yield an extra piece to stash in the freezer, and the pots of oatmeal and quinoa make double batches (also freezable). Before you shop for weeks two and three, do a quick scan to see what's already good to go!

## Produce

- ✓ Blueberries (1 cup)
- ✓ Raspberries (½ cup)

- ✓ Blackberries (½ cup)
- ✓ 1 mango, plus more for snacks if using
- ✓ 1 orange (for Citrus Dressing)
- ✓ 1 apple, for snacks
- ✓ 8 to 10 limes
- ✓ 4 to 6 lemons
- ✓ 1 avocado, for snacks
- ✓ 1 bag romaine hearts
- ✓ 1 head Boston or bibb lettuce
- ✓ 2 (5-oz) packages baby spinach
- ✓ 1 (5-oz) package baby arugula
- ✓ 1 head red cabbage
- ✓ 2 pints grape tomatoes, plus more for snacks if using
- ✓ 1 head broccoli (4 cups florets)
- ✓ 1 head cauliflower (4 cups florets)
- ✓ 4 red bell peppers
- ✓ 2 bell peppers, any color
- ✓ 2 zucchini
- ✓ 1 English cucumber, plus more for snacks if using
- ✓ 1 head celery

- ✓ 1 bunch radishes
- ✓ 1 package presliced white mushrooms (1½ cups)
- ✓ 1 hand ginger
- ✓ 2 heads garlic
- ✓ 6 to 8 onions
- ✓ 1 bunch scallions
- ✓ Herbs: mint, rosemary, thyme, and cilantro (1 bunch each)

## Dairy

- ✓ 2% milk (1½ cups)
- ✓ 1% milk or soy milk (3 cups)
- ✓ Plain 2% Greek yogurt (2 cups)

## Meat, Fish And Soy Proteins

- ✓ 2 (4-oz) boneless skinless chicken breasts
- ✓ 2 (4-oz) skinless salmon fillets
- ✓ 1 (8-oz) package soy tempeh
- ✓ 1 (14-oz) package extra-firm tofu
- ✓ 1 lb. silken soft tofu

# Grocery Items

- ✓ 1 (14.5-oz) can no-salt-added diced tomatoes
- ✓ 1 can chipotle chile in adobo
- ✓ 1 (13.5-oz) can light coconut milk
- ✓ 1 package mini whole-grain pita rounds
- ✓ 7 (15.5-oz) cans low sodium black beans
- ✓ Capers
- ✓ Quinoa (1⅓ cups)
- ✓ Steel-cut oatmeal (1 cup)
- ✓ Hummus, for snacks
- ✓ Nut butter, for snacks

# Oils, Vinegar And Condiments

- ✓ Extra-virgin olive oil
- ✓ Toasted sesame oil
- ✓ Balsamic vinegar
- ✓ Red wine vinegar
- ✓ Reduced-sodium tamari
- ✓ Dijon mustard

✓ Green curry paste (Look for this in the international or Asian foods aisle.)

## Spices

✓ Chili powder
✓ Dried thyme
✓ Ground cumin
✓ Nutmeg
✓ Cinnamon stick
✓ Pure vanilla extract

## Nuts And Seeds

✓ Almonds, for snacks
✓ Pumpkin seeds
✓ Sunflower seeds
✓ Walnuts

## Wednesday Prep

You'll need to refresh your fruit and veggie stash for the second half of the week, but check the crisper before you shop there might be some leftovers that can assist.

## Produce

- ✓ Blueberries (1 cup)
- ✓ Raspberries (½ cup)
- ✓ Blackberries (½ cup)
- ✓ 1 mango
- ✓ Mixed greens
- ✓ 1 bag romaine hearts
- ✓ 1 (5-oz) package baby spinach
- ✓ 1 avocado
- ✓ 1 pint grape tomatoes
- ✓ 1 English cucumber
- ✓ 2 red bell peppers
- ✓ Cauliflower (3 cups florets)
- ✓ 3 limes
- ✓ 3 lemons
- ✓ Herbs: basil, cilantro, mint

# THE 15 BEST WEIGHT-LOSS RECIPES YOU CAN MAKE IN 30 MINUTES OR LESS

## Thai Steak Salad.

Steak lovers rejoiced in 2015 when research in the International Journal of Obesity proclaimed the high-protein diet was the winner of weight-loss diets. The conclusion: Increasing your protein, dropping your carbs slightly, and focusing on getting higher quality carbohydrates like whole grains and produce helps you lose weight and keep it off. Thats' where this fresh-tasting weight-loss recipe for Thai steak salad by celebrity Food Network chef Ellie Krieger comes in. It's brightly flavored with lime juice, ginger, basil, and cilantro, and once the meat is marinated, and it comes together in just half an hour. Learn 12 more diet secrets of people who maintained their weight loss.

# Red Beans And Coconut Rice

Forget complicated, expensive diet plans (which don't work anyway) and just focus on fiber, suggests an recent study published in the Annals of Internal Medicine. The findings indicate that making just one dietary change setting a goal of eating 30 grams of fiber each day can help you lose weight, lower your blood pressure, and improve your body's response to insulin. As, a shortcut, make a meal of rice and beans, which provides a bowlful of plant-based protein (20 to 25 grams) and fiber (about 15 grams). Beans and rice don't have to be boring! Make this simply delicious 30-minute island-inspired coconut rice and beans recipe from epicurious.com, using light coconut milk.

# Green Tea Smoothie

You know green tea is good for you because of all its antioxidants, but the combo of caffeine and the free radical-fighting catechin EGCG in green tea has been found to help people lose weight and keep it off, according to an meta-analysis of 11 studies in the International Journal of Obesity. If you're looking for a cool alternative, try this creamy low-carb green tea smoothie made with matcha.

# Red Lentil Soup

Eating soup is one of the simplest, pain-free ways to drop a size and shed belly fat. In this study from Pennsylvania State University, participants who ate soup before consuming a lunch entrée ended up downing 20 percent fewer calories overall than people who skipped soup. Adding vegetables and protein to your soup also helps keep you fuller longer, so you'll be less hungry later on. This weight-loss recipe for red lentil soup has a whopping 13 grams of protein per cup and is ready in 25 minutes. Sauté a teaspoon or two of fresh, grated ginger with the onion and add a pinch of cayenne for an extra flavor boost.

## Tzatziki

Dunk it, dzrizzle it, szlather it no matter what you do with Greek tzatziki, it tastes wonderful. Hard to believe this special sauce is made of just Greek yogurt, cucumbers, garlic, and seasonings it can transform grilled fish and meat, simple crudités, or a veggie- and lentil-filled pita into an fantastic meal. We love this tzatziki recipe with lemon zest and dill from foodnetwork.com. Yogurt can be a key ingredient to any successful diet, as it helps you drop pounds and trim your waistline. Most experts point to the yogurt's generous amount of protein (about 18 grams per serving) for helping you feel full and satisfied, but the active cultures also could help shed body fat by correcting your gut bacteria. Find out how to pick the best probiotics for weight loss.

## Farmers Market Quinoa Salad

How do I love thee, quinoa? Let me count the ways: One, you have almost twice the protein of brown rice; two, your chewy texture and nutty flavor make everything else in the bowl taste better; and three, all that protein and fiber, along with healthy fats and a small dose of carbs, keep my blood sugar steady. Better yet, you cook faster than a pot of rice quinoa is ready in about 15 minutes. For, a quick weight-loss recipe, throw together this farmers market quinoa salad.

## Super Seedy Granola Bars

The itsy-bitsy super seeds chia and flax are tiny nutritional powerhouses. They have omega-3 (particularly alpha-linolenic acid) and omega-6 fatty acids, protein, fiber, flavonoids, a host of vitamins and minerals—not to mention great flavor and crunch. In research, the seeds increase a sense of fullness while reducing appetite. And what better way to enjoy them than combined with dates, sunflower and hemp seeds, and nuts for the ultimate homemade granola bar? Check out these easy super seedy granola bars from minimalistbaker.com.

## Fried Cauliflower Rice

Researchers have found that boosting your intake of clean, fiber-rich veggies is one of the smartest ways to slim and trim your body. A simple way to accomplish this is to make an easy Chinese stir-fried vegetable rice using prepared (or homemade) cauliflower rice as the base. We're crazy about this flexible-ingredient 15-minute fried cauliflower rice recipe from pinchofyum.com, which has eggs and tofu for protein. Follow the weight-loss recipe verbatim, or add seasonal vegetables and herbs you already have in the crisper.

## Yogurt-Marinated Chicken Kebabs

Pure protein marinated in a spicy yogurt sauce to keep it tender and juicy is what weight-loss dreams are made of. Skewering lean chicken or steak tenders is a great way to prepare healthy food fast. This recipe for spicy chicken kebabs from cookbook author Steven Raichland calls for an overnight marinade, but your hands-on time is only about 15 minutes. If you don't have a grill, you can broil them in your oven. With mouthwatering weight-loss recipes like this, you'll forget you're on a diet..

## Nicoise Salad

One thing French women know is how to make the perfect diet plate. Take Nicoise salad: a couple of cans of tuna (in olive oil is best), hard-cooked egg, steamed green beans, tomatoes, and olives, dressed with vinaigrette.

It's heaven on a plate that just happens to be loaded with protein, fiber, and healthy fats. To serve the salad chilled, prep it early or the day before. Martha Stewart makes an mean Nicoise salad you'll want to make again and again. Note: Your best choice for seafood is chunk light tuna, which comes from the smaller skipjack or yellowfin and has less mercury than canned white albacore tuna.

## No-Bake Vegan Chocolate Tart

Chocolate lovers, let go of your guilt: Unsweetened cocoa powder has about two grams of fiber per tablespoon, plus iron, manganese, magnesium, and zinc. Cocoa also has high flavonoid content, so it lowers your risk of diabetes and heart disease. If you're craving chocolate, go ahead and add some cocoa powder to your protein shake. Or if a little won't do, try this deep, dark raw vegan chocolate tart from food52.com whipped up with cocoa, avocados, and coconut oil.

## Cauliflower And Kale Frittata

This low-cal cauliflower and kale frittata recipe takes just 20 minutes to make and packs a one-two punch of protein and fiber that will keep you satisfied and energized all day. Inspired by a traditional Spanish tortilla (typically studded with starchy potatoes), this healthier frittata has less than 300 calories for an large wedge by swapping in low-carb cauliflower. Serve it with a crisp arugula and radish salad dressed with extra virgin olive oil and lemon juice.

## Ready-To-Eat Berry Parfaits

Healthy food that's quick and convenient means you're more likely to eat it and stay on a sensible diet plan (as opposed to diving into the box of donuts in the breakroom). You can't beat the idea of packing superfoods like berries in jars for nutrient-rich snacks and lunches that you can grab and go with. Layer sliced berries with thick Greek yogurt and maple syrup (or your preferred natural sweetener) in an Mason jar.

# Savory Vegetable Smoothie .

Left glass of green vegetable smoothie near ingredients celery, avocado, cucumber, apple, kiwi and herbs, right empty space on wooden background. Green vegetable smoothie and ingredients. Horizontal.

Who says all smoothies have to be sweet? Make a savory one and keep it filling by adding power nutrients and fiber. This vegan smoothie from healthyblenderrecipes.com is packed with vegetables, coconut water, olive oil, and sea salt (you can substitute kosher salt). Non-vegans can pump up the protein with ancientnutrition.com's Bone Broth Protein Greens, which is rich in collagen, gelatin, glucosamine, chondroitin, and hyaluronic acid to support healthy skin, nails, and joints.

# CONCLUSION.

PCOS is one of the most common disorders affecting women of reproductive age. As a syndrome, it has multiple components, including breeding, metabolic, and cardiovascular, with long-term health concerns that cross the life span.

Although not well understood, insulin resistance seems to underlie many of the clinical manifestations of PCOS. Insulin resistance also appears to increase the risk of glucose intolerance, type 2 diabetes, and lipid abnormalities.

Treatment of this disorder should focus on reduction of androgen-associated symptoms, the protection of the endometrium, and reduction of the long-term risks of diabetes and cardiovascular complications.

For many women with this syndrome,improving infertility is a primary goal of therapy. Nurse-midwives can assess and manage many of the presenting complaints and lifestyle issues, such as menstrual disorders, hirsutism, and obesity, which are associated with PCOS. A nurse may choose to manage the more complex problems, such as infertility and insulin resistance. We must act to prevent the far-reaching consequences of this syndrome.

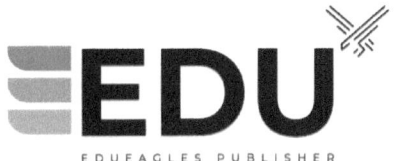